Last Minute Picture Tests for MRCP 2

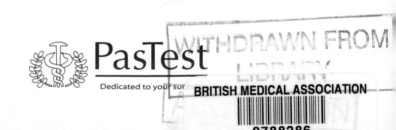

PasTest

Dedicated to your success

Last Minute Picture Tests for MRCP 2

W Stephen Waring BMedSci MRCP (UK) PhD

Consultant Physician & Honorary Senior Lecturer
Scottish Poisons Information Bureau
Royal Infirmary of Edinburgh
Edinburgh

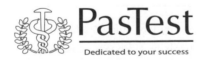

PasTest
Dedicated to your success

© 2006 PASTEST LTD
Egerton Court
Parkgate Estate
Knutsford
Cheshire
WA16 8DX

Telephone: 01565 752000

First Published 2006

ISBN: 1 904627 78 1

A catalogue record for this book is available from the British Library.

The information contained within this book was obtained by the author from
reliable sources. However, while every effort has been made to ensure its accuracy,
no responsibility for loss, damage or injury occasioned to any person acting or
refraining from action as a result of information contained herein can be accepted
by the publishers or author.

PasTest Revision Books and Intensive Courses

PasTest has been established in the field of postgraduate medical education
since 1972, providing revision books and intensive study courses for doctors
preparing for their professional examinations.

Books and courses are available for the following specialties:

MRCGP, MRCP Parts 1 and 2, MRCPCH Parts 1 and 2, MRCPsych, MRCS,
MRCOG Parts 1 and 2, DRCOG, DCH, FRCA, PLAB Parts 1 and 2.

For further details contact:

PasTest, Freepost, Knutsford, Cheshire WA16 7BR

Tel: 01565 752000   **Fax: 01565 650264**
www.pastest.co.uk   **enquiries@pastest.co.uk**

Text typeset and designed by Type Study, Scarborough, North Yorkshire

Printed and bound in the UK by Alden Press, Oxfordshire

CONTENTS

CONTRIBUTORS

Alice Miller MA MBChB
Senior House Officer in Medicine, Royal Infirmary of Edinburgh, Edinburgh

We acknowledge the contribution given by a colleague based at St John's Hospital, Livingston.

INTRODUCTION

The MRCP(UK) diploma is a recognised entry qualification for higher specialist training in medicine and its related specialties. Eligibility for the MRCP(UK) diploma normally requires candidates to successfully complete the MRCP(UK) examination, which has two parts involving three separate assessments; the Part 1 examination, the Part 2 written examination, and the Part 2 clinical examination. Candidates can undertake the Part 2 written examination if they have successfully completed the Part 1 examination, or if they have exemption from the Part 1 examination. The MRCP(UK) Part 2 written examination is overseen by administrative offices in Edinburgh, Glasgow and London, and can be undertaken at any one of several established UK centres, or at one of a growing number of overseas centres.

The format of the exam is constantly changing to reflect new patterns of teaching methods, and advances in knowledge and skills required for current clinical practice. From December 2005 onwards, the examination has been delivered as three 3-hour written papers over the course of two days: Papers 1&2 on one day, and Paper 3 on the next day. Questions involve a 'best of five' format (one correct answer selected from five possible options), and an 'n of many' format (two or three correct answers selected from ten to fifteen possible options). 'Negative marking' has been phased out so that in the current Part 2 written examination, a correct answer will score +1, whereas no attempt or an incorrect answer will score 0. These changes have been taken to create a more reliable assessment of candidate's abilities.

The Part 2 written examination is designed to assess candidates' knowledge about diagnosis, investigation, management, and prognosis in relation to important diseases. Inclusion of contextual clinical scenarios aims to keep the exam relevant to everyday practice. The questions may include the results of investigations, and may be accompanied by illustrative material such as clinical photographs, ECG traces, radiographic images or microscopic appearances. Each of the three papers in the MRCP(UK) Part 2 written examination contains around 100 questions. The exam is criterion referenced, and a pass mark is set before each diet by experienced clinicians responsible for standard setting. Questions are chosen to represent each of the main clinical specialties in the following proportions:

Specialties

Neurology, ophthalmology, psychiatry	11%
Cardiology	10%
Clinical pharmacology & toxicology	10%
Endocrinology & metabolic medicine	10%
Gastroenterology	10%
Renal medicine	10%
Respiratory medicine	10%
Infectious diseases, tropical medicine & STDs	9%
Rheumatology	6%
Clinical haematology & immunology	5%
Oncology & palliative medicine	5%
Dermatology	4%

This book contains 150 colour illustrations that cover a wide range of clinical conditions. The photographs include radiographs, blood films, ECG traces, pathological examples and other formats. They are accompanied by questions that are in the same style as is commonly encountered in the exam itself, and give a certain amount of relevant history to help the candidate make the most appropriate diagnosis. The answers are succinct and should aid the candidate in revision. *Last Minute Picture Tests for MRCP* gives candidates an opportunity to refresh their knowledge over a broad range of topics included in the exam syllabus. The answers are given as an *aide memoir* rather than an exhaustive summary of individual topics, to allow candidates to cover large numbers of questions more quickly. Explanations are given for certain modalities of investigation that might be unfamiliar to some candidates, for example echocardiography.

Useful websites for further information are:

1. http://www.mrcpuk.org/plain/mrcppt2.html
   Further information on the MRCP Part 2 written exam regulations and application process.
2. http://www.pastestonline.co.uk/
   Online revision source with practice papers (different questions from those appearing in the book range), including a free demo.

Good luck!

WSW
2006

QUESTIONS

1. The following abdominal ultrasound scan with Doppler flow was performed in a 56-year-old patient with established peripheral vascular disease. What is the most likely diagnosis?

- A   Abdominal aortic aneurysm
- B   Aortic dissection
- C   Arterio-venous malformation
- D   Polyarteritis nodosa
- E   Renal artery stenosis

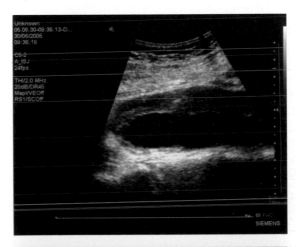

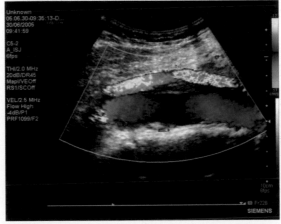

Answer on p. 4

1

2.   A 45-year-old woman attends the A&E department complaining of severe anterior chest wall pain, associated with vomiting. Which of the following diagnoses does the ECG appearance most strongly suggest?

☐ **A**   Acute anterior myocardial infarction

☐ **B**   Acute inferolateral myocardial infarction

☐ **C**   Acute pulmonary embolism

☐ **D**   Dissection of the ascending aorta

☐ **E**   Right ventricular infarction

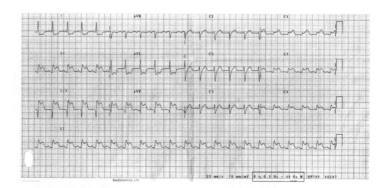

3. This 61-year-old man has been admitted to hospital due to recurrent falls and poor mobility. You are asked to review him because he is complaining of deterioration of his vision. What is the most likely diagnosis?

- [ ] **A** Central retinal artery occlusion
- [ ] **B** Central retinal vein occlusion
- [ ] **C** CMV retinitis
- [ ] **D** Grade IV hypertensive retinopathy
- [ ] **E** Polyarteritis nodosa

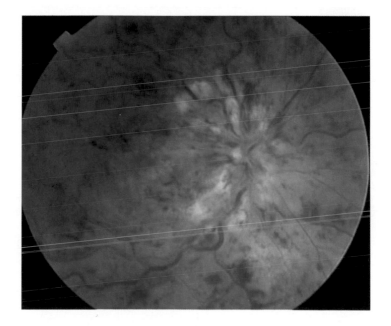

Answer on p. 4

1. B: Aortic dissection

The scan shows a longitudinal tear along the aorta with laminar flow in the main aortic lumen (shown in blue to red) and turbulent flow within the dissection (scattered red, blue, yellow). Aortic dissection involves the ascending aorta in 70% of cases, descending aorta in 20% and the aortic arch in 10%. Abdominal aortic aneurysm dissection usually occurs at or below the renal artery level, and most commonly in patients with aortic aneurysm.

2. B: Acute inferolateral myocardial infarction

Significant ST segment elevation is seen in both inferior (II, III and aVF) and lateral leads (V4–6). This is likely to represent occlusion of the left anterior descending coronary artery, but there is insufficient information to suggest underlying aortic dissection.

3. B: Central retinal vein occlusion

There are extensive retinal haemorrhages and exudates; all sectors of the retina are involved, in contrast to the pattern seen in branch retinal vein occlusion. Central retinal vein occlusion is a thrombotic disorder (in contrast to central retinal artery occlusion, which is usually embolic in origin). Risk factors are glaucoma and raised intraocular pressure.

4. A 51-year-old woman is undergoing investigation of iron-deficiency anaemia. The following shows a barium enema investigation. What is the most likely explanation of the anaemia?

- **A** Ascending colon carcinoma
- **B** Collagenous colitis
- **C** Ischaemic colitis
- **D** Sigmoid carcinoma
- **E** Ulcerative colitis

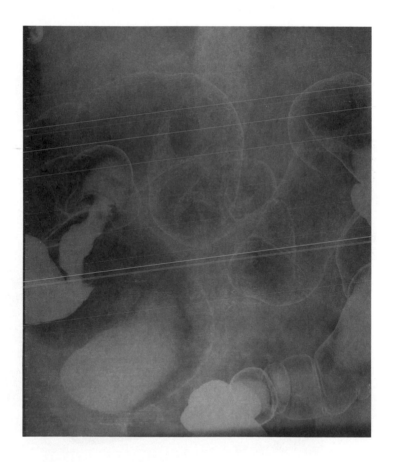

Answer on p. 8

5. A 43-year-old man is admitted after a deliberate overdose of paracetamol and is commenced on an *N*-acetylcysteine (NAC) infusion. Twenty minutes later, he complains of nausea and is found to have a heart rate of 102 beats per minute and blood pressure 106/48 mmHg. What mechanism is thought most likely to be responsible for this adverse reaction?

A   Alpha-adrenergic receptor activation

B   Beta-2 receptor stimulation

C   Histamine-1 receptor stimulation

D   Increased vagal tone

E   Muscarinic receptor activation

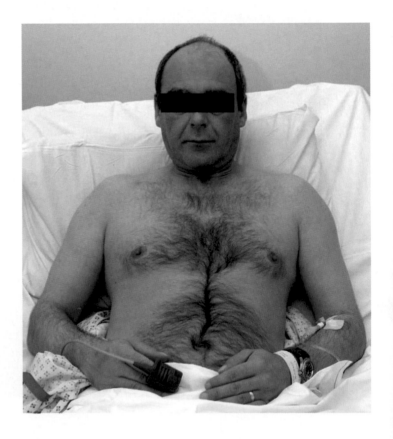

Answer on p. 8

6. This 55-year-old woman is undergoing investigation of unexplained anaemia. Her haemoglobin is 9.8 g/dl and mean cell volume 118 fl. What is the most likely explanation for her anaemia?

- A Coeliac disease
- B Pernicious anaemia
- C Malnutrition
- D Thalassaemia
- E Ulcerative colitis

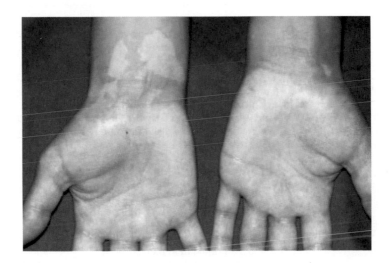

Answer on p. 8

4.   **A: Ascending colon carcinoma**

Narrowing of the lumen affecting the ascending colon, giving rise to characteristic 'apple-core' appearance. Carcinoma of the caecum and ascending colon often presents with iron-deficiency anaemia. Sensitivity for polyp and carcinoma detection is around 80% for double-contrast barium enema versus 90% for colonoscopy, although sensitivity is similar for large lesions. CT colonography (virtual colonoscopy) is less sensitive but may be useful where patients are unable to tolerate barium enema or colonoscopy.

5.   **C: Histamine-1 receptor stimulation**

Anaphylactoid reactions are a recognised adverse effect of NAC and occur in around 10–15% of patients, usually within 30 minutes after commencing treatment. Features include histamine-mediated flushing and vasodilatation (as shown). Temporary discontinuation of infusion is usually sufficient to allow resolution of effects, although antihistamine treatment may be required.

6.   **B: Pernicious anaemia**

Vitiligo is an autoimmune disorder mediated by autoantibodies that target melanocytes resulting in patches of hypopigmentation. Patients are at increased risk of sunburn and skin cancer at affected sites in sun-exposed areas. It is associated with other autoimmune disorders including Grave's disease, hypoparathyroidism, insulin-dependent diabetes mellitus, Addison's disease and primary ovarian failure.

7. This 55-year-old woman is under regular review in the cardiovascular risk clinic, and is receiving treatment for hypertension and hypercholesterolaemia. Which one of her medications is most likely to have caused this adverse effect?

- ☐ **A** Atenolol
- ☐ **B** Clopidogrel
- ☐ **C** Lisinopril
- ☐ **D** Nifedipine
- ☐ **E** Simvastatin

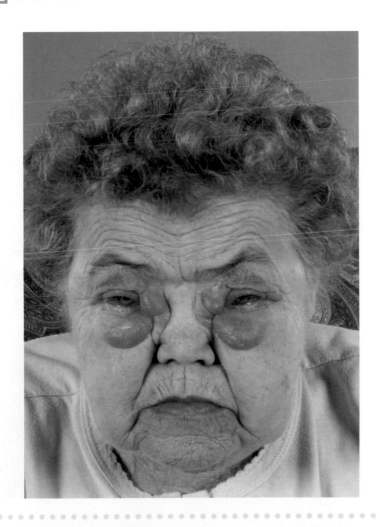

Answer on p. 12

8. A 61-year-old man is found to have a mass in the upper abdomen, and is referred for abdominal ultrasound scan with Doppler flow. Which one of the following complications is most likely to arise from this disorder?

- A Acute ischaemic stroke
- B Ankle oedema
- C Digital embolisation affecting the toes
- D Disseminated intravascular coagulation
- E Splinter nailbed haemorrhages

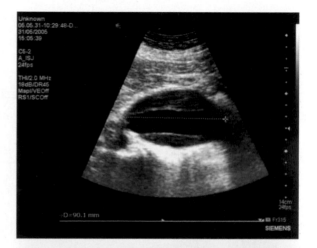

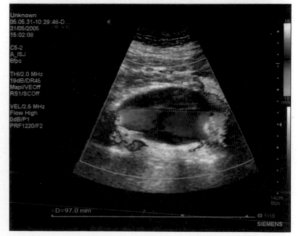

Answer on p. 12

9. This is the forearm of a 54-year-old woman who attends clinic for routine review of her longstanding joint disease. What is the most likely implication of the abnormality noted on her forearm?

- [ ] **A** Abnormal renal urate clearance
- [ ] **B** Higher risk of ischaemic heart disease
- [ ] **C** Multiple endocrine neoplasia
- [ ] **D** Positive for anti-IgG IgM antibody
- [ ] **E** Systemic inflammation

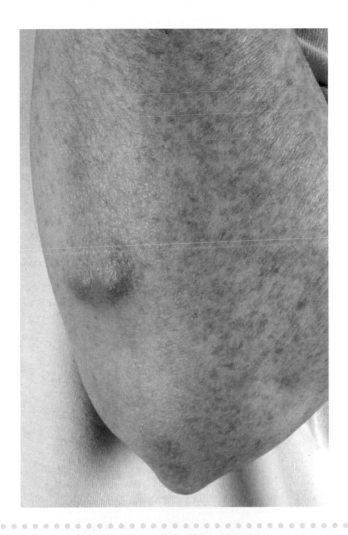

Answer on p. 12

| 7. | **C: Lisinopril** |

Angioedema is a rare but potentially serious adverse event of angiotensin-converting enzyme inhibitor therapy that occurs in between 0.5% and 1.0% of patients. Risk factors are Afro-Caribbean race, age more than 65 years and a history of atopy. It usually occurs shortly after initiation, but can occur at any time.

| 8. | **C: Digital embolisation affecting the toes** |

The scan demonstrates a large abdominal aortic aneurysm. There is clot within the dilated walls of the aneurysm, and laminar blood flow within the central portion of the vessel. Other recognised complications are back pain, dissection and rupture. Women >65 years age, significant smoking history and aneurysm diameter >5.5 cm diameter significantly increase risk of rupture.

| 9. | **D: Positive for anti-Ig IgM antibody** |

Rheumatoid nodules are subcutaneous or intradermal nodules that are typically hard and painless. They can develop within various organs, particularly the lungs, and arthralgia is the main joint symptom. Their presence is associated with a high likelihood of rheumatoid factor positivity. Rheumatoid nodulosis is a specific disorder requiring all of: (1) multiple subcutaneous rheumatoid nodules, (2) recurrent joint symptoms with minimal radiographic damage, (3) a benign course and (4) no significant systemic manifestations.

10. This 23-year-old man with type 1 diabetes mellitus complains of a painful rash overlying both lower limbs during a routine follow-up clinic appointment. What is the most likely explanation?

☐ **A** Erythema multiforme

☐ **B** Erythema nodosum

☐ **C** Henoch–Schönlein purpura

☐ **D** Necrobiosis lipoidica

☐ **E** Pyoderma gangrenosum

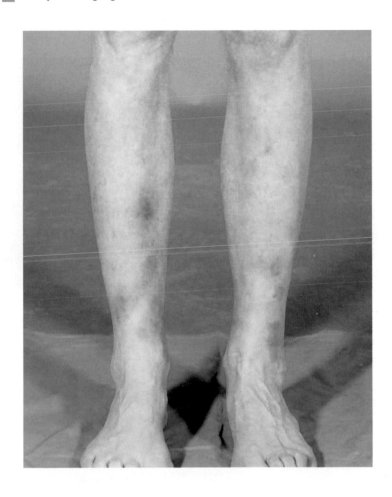

11. This 56-year-old man has experienced a number of episodes of dizziness associated with transient left-sided arm weakness. He is referred for echocardiography. Which one of the following diagnoses is most likely based on the two-dimensional images shown?

    A Atrial septal defect

    B Hypertrophic cardiomyopathy

    C Left atrial thrombus

    D Pericardial effusion

    E Ventricular aneurysm

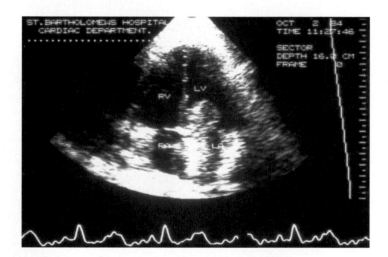

Answer on p. 16

12. A 65-year-old man is admitted to the acute medical admissions unit after a collapse associated with transient loss of consciousness. His admission ECG is shown below. Which of the following statements best describes the rhythm shown?

- A Complete heart block
- B DDD pacemaker functioning normally
- C Failure of atrial sensing
- D Failure of ventricular inhibiting
- E Failure of ventricular sensing

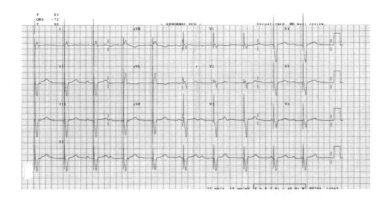

10. **B: Erythema nodosum**

Erythema nodosum is a panniculitis of uncertain aetiology that may occur as an isolated phenomenon or in association with a number of underlying disorders including Behçet's disease, cat scratch disease, infectious mononucleosis, inflammatory bowel disease, tuberculosis, sarcoidosis and streptococcal respiratory tract infection. Tuberculosis, *Yersinia*, chlamydia and hepatitis B are rare causes. It is also associated with drugs including the combined oral contraceptive pill, penicillin and sulfonamides.

11. **C: Left atrial thrombus**

There is abnormally high echogenicity (white) within the left atrium (lower right), with extension into the left ventricle across the mitral valve. This appearance is more typically associated with left atrial myxomata that, although rare, adhere more firmly than thrombus. Extensive thrombus can extend from the left atrial appendage, and may be associated with recurrent thromboembolism.

12. **A: Complete heart block**

Atrial electrical activity is not followed directly by QRS complex activity or ventricular pacing. With a functioning DDD pacemaker, ventricular pacing would be triggered within a pre-specified time after atrial depolarisation (and inhibited by intrinsic ventricular electrical activity within this period). The rhythm strip suggests a VVI pacemaker with rate set to 60/min (no intrinsic ventricular complexes occurred, so the inhibiting function cannot be fully assessed from this ECG).

13. This 58-year-old woman presented via the A&E department with a 6-month history of progressive breathlessness. What underlying diagnosis is most likely to account for these abnormalities?

- [ ] **A** Amyloidosis
- [ ] **B** Congestive heart failure
- [ ] **C** Nephrotic syndrome
- [ ] **D** Protein malabsorption
- [ ] **E** Yellow nail syndrome

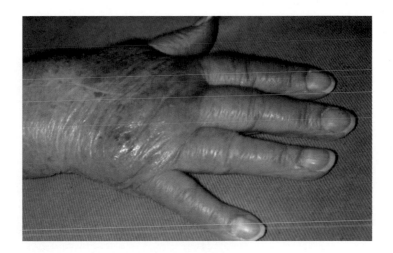

14. A 34-year-old man is referred for investigation of dry cough and fever associated with haemoptysis. Cardiac auscultation is normal, peripheral pulses are intact and peripheral oedema is absent. Respiratory examination reveals end-inspiratory crackles overlying the middle and lower zones of both lung fields. What is the most likely underlying diagnosis?

A Allergic bronchopulmonary aspergillosis

B Severe streptococcal pneumonia

C *Pneumocystis carinii* pneumonia

D Tuberculosis

E Wegener's granulomatosis

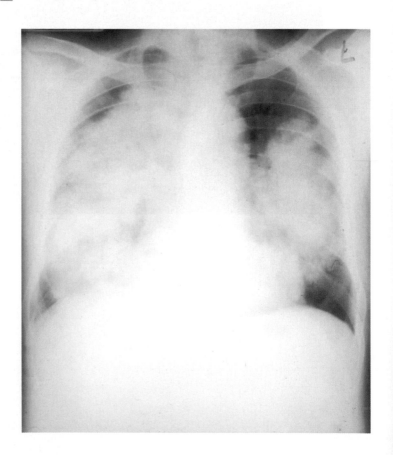

Answer on p. 20

15. This 56-year-old man is undergoing investigation of progressive weight loss over the past year, associated with altered bowel habit and deranged liver biochemistry tests. What is the most likely underlying diagnosis?

☐ **A** Addision's disease

☐ **B** Chronic pancreatitis

☐ **C** Coeliac disease

☐ **D** Haemochromatosis

☐ **E** Tuberculosis

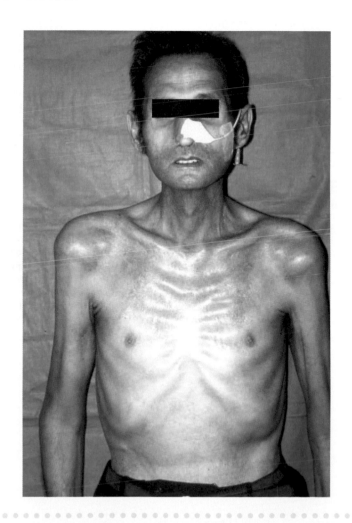

13. **C: Nephrotic syndrome**

Leuconychia indicates hypoalbuminaemia, and there is peripheral oedema involving the hand. Characteristic features of nephrotic syndrome include heavy proteinuria (typically >3g/day), hypoalbuminaemia, hypercholesterolaemia and peripheral oedema. Protein malabsorption is rarely so severe as to result in profound hypoalbuminaemia.

14. **E: Wegener's granulomatosis**

The chest radiograph appearances of pulmonary haemorrhage can mimic those of pulmonary oedema and pneumonia. Wegener's granulomatosis is characterised by a granulomatous small vessel vasculitis that primarily involves the nasopharynx, lungs and kidney, and can be confirmed by demonstration of non-caseating granulomata on biopsy, and positive immunofluorescence cANCA antibody test.

15. **D: Haemochromatosis**

Generalised hyperpigmentation is seen, involving non-sun exposed areas. Hereditary haemochromatosis is a disorder of iron metabolism characterised by a progressive tissue iron overload and irreversible organ damage if untreated; chronic pancreatitis is a recognised complication. Elevated transferrin saturation and serum ferritin are used in establishing the diagnosis, and phlebotomy is the mainstay of treatment. Outcome is very good if phlebotomy is started before significant organ damage occurs.

16. This 48-year-old lady is referred to the hypertension clinic by her GP, having been found to have blood pressures of 152/100 mmHg, 156/92 mmHg and 158/96 mmHg during three separate visits. What is shown on retinal examination?

- A Accelerated hypertension
- B Non-proliferative diabetic retinopathy
- C Proliferative diabetic retinopathy
- D Grade III hypertensive retinopathy
- E Grade IV hypertensive retinopathy

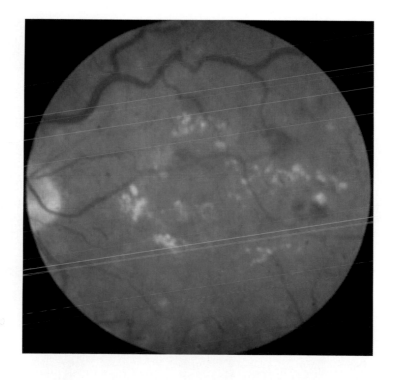

17. This elderly patient is asymptomatic, and has been referred to the hypertension clinic with isolated systolic hypertension. Which one of the following diagnoses is most likely to account for the appearance of his lower limbs?

- A   Childhood rickets
- B   Hyperparathyroidism
- C   Metastatic breast cancer
- D   Multiple myeloma
- E   Previous trauma

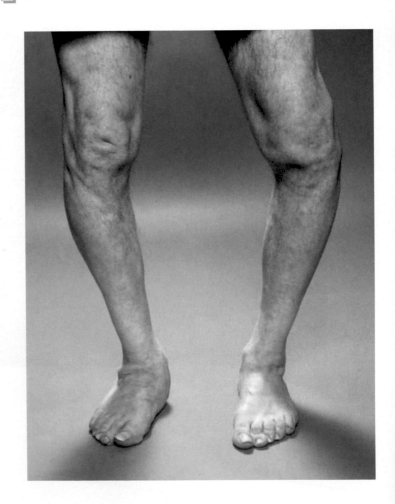

18. This 34-year-old man is referred by his GP to the DVT clinic for assessment of swelling in the lower limb. He is normally fit and active, and plays racquet sports regularly. The leg is shown from posterior and posterolateral aspects. What is the most likely cause?

- A Arterio-venous malformation
- B Leiomyoma
- C Neurofibroma
- D Popliteal cyst
- E Ruptured Baker's cyst

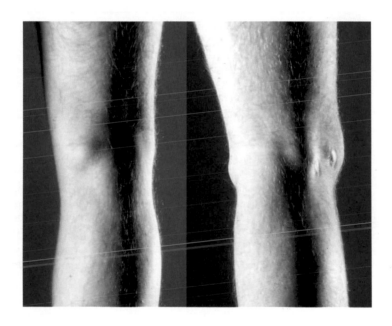

16. **B: Non-proliferative diabetic retinopathy**

Characteristic appearance of microaneurysms (difficult to distinguish from dot haemorrhages), retinal haemorrhages and hard exudates that arise from increased capillary permeability and leakage of serum lipids and proteins. Patients with diabetes and co-existent hypertension are more likely to develop more severe diabetic retinopathy, which progresses more rapidly. Diffuse macular oedema is more common in patients with both diabetes and hypertension.

17. **A: Childhood rickets**

Childhood rickets is now uncommon in developed nations, but results in a typical valgus deformity that tends to persist through adulthood. Other recognised causes are Paget's bone disease and, less commonly, previous trauma with aberrant healing.

18. **D: Popliteal cyst**

Popliteal cyst, also known as a Baker's cyst, is a discrete swelling that is typically painless. Normally, there is no significant underlying pathology and they often resolve spontaneously. Rupture of the cyst can result in local pain and inflammation tracking distally, which can mimic deep vein thrombosis.

19. This 34-year-old man is under regular cardiology review. What is the most likely underlying diagnosis?

☐ **A** Alport's syndrome

☐ **B** Benign joint hypermobility syndrome

☐ **C** Homocysteinaemia

☐ **D** Marfan's syndrome

☐ **E** Relapsing polychondritis

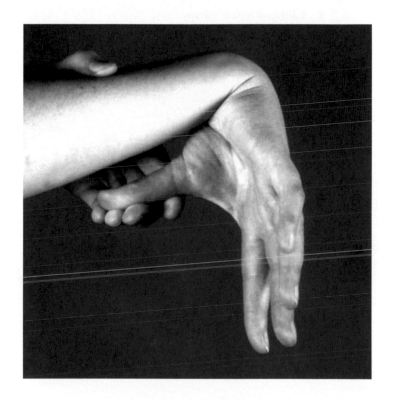

20. A 48-year-old lifelong smoker is rushed to the coronary care unit 1 hour after sudden onset of severe chest pain, sweating and nausea. Taking into account the ECG abnormalities, which of these immediate treatments is most likely to improve survival?

A   High-flow oxygen administration

B   Intravenous beta-blocker administration

C   Intravenous t-PA

D   Subcutaneous heparin administration

E   Sublingual nitrate therapy

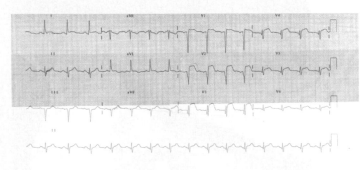

Answer on p. 28

21. This 64-year-old retired coal-miner presents with progressive breathlessness on exertion. What diagnosis is most likely to explain the features shown in his plain chest radiograph?

- [ ] **A** Lung collapse
- [ ] **B** Previous lung cancer
- [ ] **C** Restrictive cardiomyopathy
- [ ] **D** Severe lung fibrosis
- [ ] **E** Tension pneumothorax

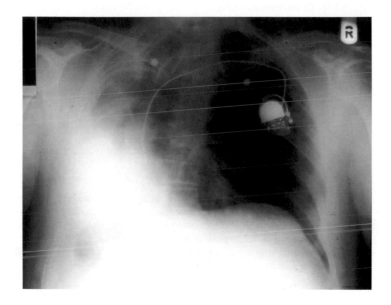

Answer on p. 28

19. **D: Marfan's syndrome**

Joint hypermobility is common in some healthy young patients, and those with rare hereditary connective tissue disorders including Ehlers–Danlos and Marfan's syndromes, and osteogenesis imperfecta. Patients with symptoms attributable to their joint hypermobility are said to have benign joint hypermobility syndrome.

20. **C: Intravenous t-PA**

The ECG confirms acute anterolateral myocardial infarction. Early administration of antiplatelet therapy is indicated. Angiotensin-converting enzyme inhibitor and/or beta-blocker treatment should be considered and, in selected cases, early coronary intervention. Analgesia, oxygen, nitrates and diuretic therapy are symptomatic adjuncts that do not significantly influence survival.

21. **B: Previous lung cancer**

There has previously been a left pneumonectomy and there is consequent distortion of thoracic anatomy, including upper and lower mediastinal deviation to the left side. The permanent cardiac pacemaker might prompt interest in a cardiac cause for breathlessness, but it would not explain any of the diagnoses listed in the question.

22. This 21-year-old man presented with pain in both lower limbs during weight-bearing, associated with mild localised swelling. What diagnosis is suggested by the radiograph appearances and bone biopsy microscopy?

- **A** Eosinophilic granulomata
- **B** Paget's disease
- **C** Rickets
- **D** Tuberculosis
- **E** Wegener's granulomatosis

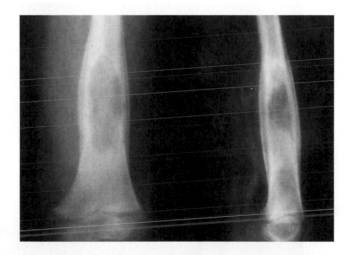

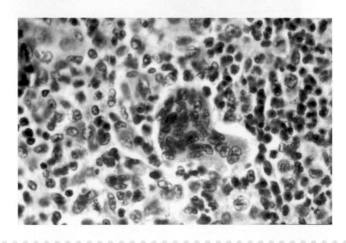

23. What is the most likely underlying explanation for the abnormal appearances seen in the foot of this previously well 52-year-old man?

- A Diabetes mellitus
- B Cerebellar degeneration
- C Lead toxicity
- D Rheumatoid arthritis
- E Tertiary syphilis

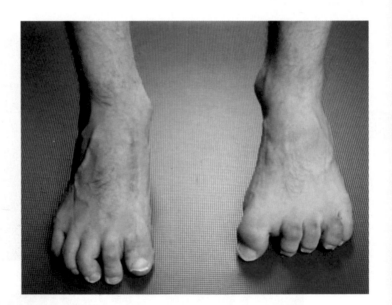

Answer on p. 32

24. Which one of the following diagnoses is most likely to account for the abnormal appearance seen in this patient's lower limbs?

☐ **A** Charcot–Marie–Tooth disease
☐ **B** Diabetes mellitus
☐ **C** Disuse atrophy
☐ **D** Leprosy
☐ **E** Syphilis

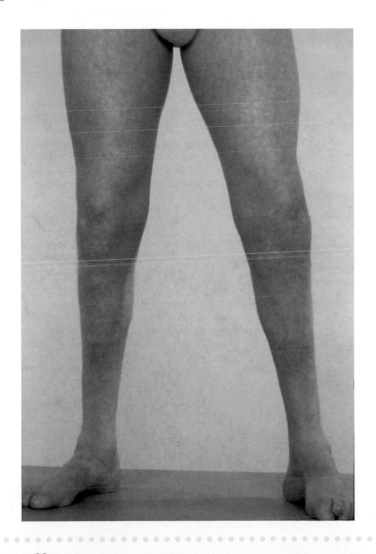

22.   **A: Eosinophilic granulomata**

Eosinophilic granuloma is a tumour-like abnormality resulting from clonal proliferation of Langerhan-type histiocytes, and typically affects children and young adults. Typical radiographic changes involve an area of radiolucency with surrounding margin of reactive bone, and histology shows Langerhan's cells with large ovoid nucleus, abundant pale staining cytoplasm and a well-defined cytoplasmic border. The lesions usually resolve spontaneously. Soft tissue and organ involvement are poor prognostic indicators, and chemotherapy or radiotherapy treatment may be required.

23.   **A: Diabetes mellitus**

This patient has clawed toes and foot associated with callosities (neuropathic claw foot or 'pes cavus'), associated with hyperextension of the metatarsal joints and flexion of the interphalangeal joints. Recognised causes include diabetes mellitus, rheumatoid arthritis, stroke, Charcot–Marie–Tooth disease, Friedreich's ataxia, neurosyphilis and subacute combined degeneration of the cord.

24.   **A: Charcot–Marie–Tooth disease**

Charcot–Marie–Tooth disease (CMT) describes a group of disorders with overlapping clinical phenotypes characterised by peripheral motor and sensory neuropathy. CMT is inherited in X-linked and autosomal recessive patterns that result in multiple mutations of genes that regulate Schwann cell and neurone function. Typical features include progressive peripheral muscle wasting over many years leading to this characteristic 'inverted champagne bottle' appearance in the lower limbs.

25. This previously well 42-year-old patient presented with fatigue and vague abdominal pain. Plain chest and abdominal radiographs are normal. What test would be best for establishing the underlying diagnosis?

A 24-hour urinary cortisol assay

B Colonoscopy

C CT abdominal scan

D Overnight dexamethasone suppression

E Short synacthen test

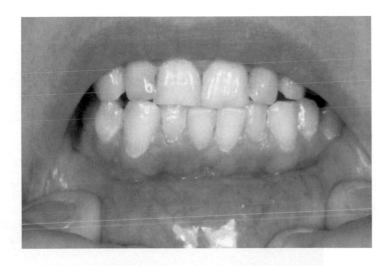

26. This echocardiogram was undertaken on a 58-year-old woman who had recently been diagnosed with a transient ischaemic attack. What two diagnoses are most likely indicated by this M-mode view?

A Aortic stenosis

B Atrial fibrillation

C Atrial myxoma

D Mitral incompetence

E Mitral stenosis

F Ventricular septal defect

G Ventricular septal hypertrophy

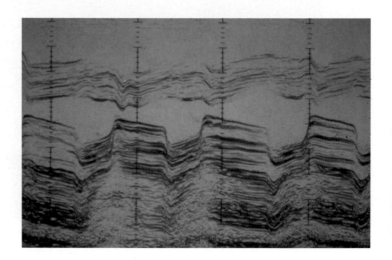

27. A 56-year-old woman is referred to the dermatology outpatient clinic for assessment of painless blisters overlying her lower limbs. On examination there is oral ulceration. What is the most likely diagnosis?

    A   Dermatitis artefacta

    B   Dermatitis herpetiformis

    C   Lymphangioma circumscriptum

    D   Pemphigoid

    E   Pemphigus

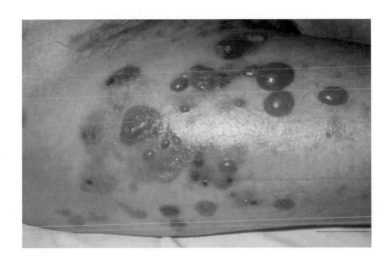

25. E: Short synacthen test

Features of Addison's disease are usually non-specific, including fatigue, nausea, abdominal pain and weight loss. Classical features are hyperpigmentation (shown in this patient's gums) and salt craving. Other features include hyperkalaemia, hyponatraemia, hypercalcaemia, anaemia and eosinophilia. Diagnosis may be confirmed by morning serum cortisol concentration <150 nmol/l and ACTH >20 pmol/l. Synacthen (tetracosactide) test is diagnostic for adrenocortical failure if serum cortisol fails to rise above 550 nmol/l.

26. B: Atrial fibrillation, E: Mitral stenosis

The mitral valve movement is restricted, with increased ECHO reflections due to reverberations and turbulent flow across the narrowed valve. The patient is in atrial fibrillation so the duration of diastole is variable, and there is loss of the normal 'a' wave in late diastole normally caused by atrial contraction. AMVL = anterior mitral valve leaflet, PMVL = posterior mitral valve leaflet, 'E' (early) wave in early diastole due to passive ventricular filling.

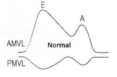
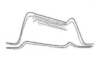
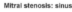

Mitral stenosis: sinus   Mitral stenosis: AF

27. E: Pemphigus

Pemphigus vulgaris is caused by autoantibodies to keratinocyte cell surface antigens resulting in acantholysis and formation of superficial blisters within the epidermis. Antibodies are found in skin biopsy in 90% of cases, which are usually IgG and less commonly IgM or IgA. There is oral involvement in 50% of cases, unlike pemphigoid. Pemphigus is fatal if left untreated, and is normally managed with topical or systemic corticosteroids; plasmapheresis, intravenous immunoglobulin and cytotoxic drugs have been used with varying success.

28. This 31-year-old patient with Hodgkin's disease attends for annual review in the Haematology Clinic. Which two of the following are the most likely causes of this appearance?

- [ ] **A** Chemotherapy-induced heart failure
- [ ] **B** Deep vein thrombosis
- [ ] **C** Femoral vein compression
- [ ] **D** Filariasis
- [ ] **E** Lymphatic obstruction
- [ ] **F** Nephrotic syndrome
- [ ] **G** Post-irradiation lymphoedema

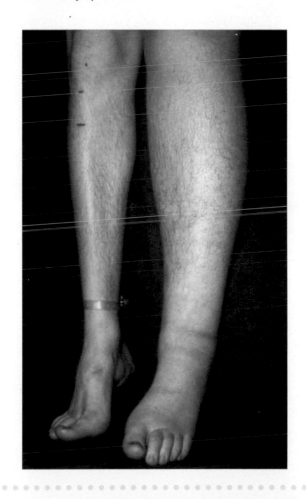

29. This lady had been referred to the dermatology outpatient clinic for assessment of a widespread rash. What is the most likely diagnosis?

☐ **A** Erythroderma

☐ **B** Erythrodermic psoriasis

☐ **C** Exfoliative dermatitis

☐ **D** Mycosis fungoides

☐ **E** Penicillin allergy

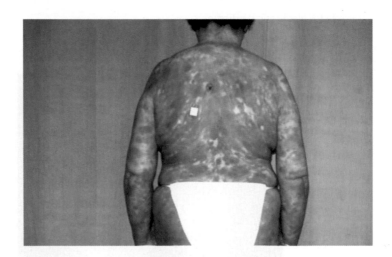

Answer on p. 40

30. This 36-year-old woman attends the diabetes outpatient department for routine follow-up. Which of the following best describes the retinal examination appearances?

   A   Diabetic maculopathy

   B   Grade III hypertensive retinopathy

   C   Mild non-proliferative diabetic retinopathy

   D   Severe non-proliferative diabetic retinopathy

   E   Mild proliferative diabetic retinopathy

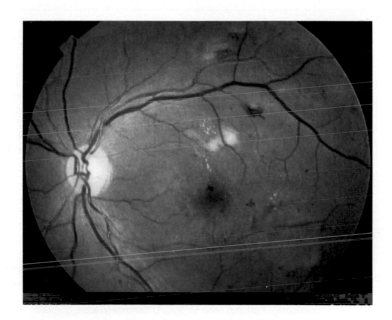

Answer on p. 40

| 28. | **E: Lymphatic obstruction, G: Post-irradiation lymphoedema** |

Peripheral oedema results from an imbalance between capillary filtration, resorption and lymphatic transport. Venous hypertension (due to valve degeneration or thrombosis) causes venous hypertension and increased filtration pressure. Primary and secondary disturbances of the lymphatic system are another important reason for interstitial liquid retention. Superficial venous distension, overlying erythema and haemosiderin pigmentation would suggest chronic venous hypertension.

| 29. | **D: Mycosis fungoides** |

Cutaneous T-cell lymphoma with manifestations in the form of patches, plaques, or cutaneous tumours. Diagnosis based on indolent clinical course and immunotyping (CD4+, CLA+, CD7 negative, and CD26 negative). Sezary syndrome is a variant characterised by diffuse erythroderma, generalised lymphadenopathy, and presence of pleomorphic circulating lymphoid cells similar to those infiltrating the skin.

| 30. | **C: Mild non-proliferative diabetic retinopathy** |

Abnormalities shown are microaneurysms, dot and blot haemorrhages, hard exudates (small, highly demarcated areas of protein and lipid accumulation), and soft exudates (larger, poorly defined 'cotton wool' spots due to nerve fibre ischaemia and oedema). Features seen in severe non-proliferative diabetic retinopathy are marked retinal ischaemia, >20 intraretinal haemorrhages in each of the 4 quadrants, and definite venous beading in ≥2 quadrants.

31. This 37-year-old woman has longstanding Crohn's disease. She is referred to the outpatient department by her GP for assessment of a rash overlying her face that has developed over the past week. What is the diagnosis?

- [ ] **A** Erysipelas
- [ ] **B** Herpes zoster
- [ ] **C** Necrobiosis lipoidica
- [ ] **D** Pyoderma gangrenosum
- [ ] **E** Pyogenic granuloma

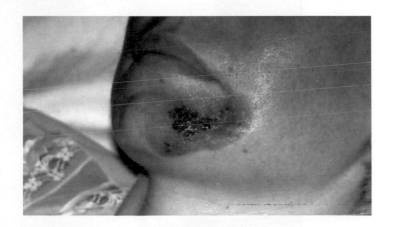

32. This 42-year-old patient is noted to have a rash overlying both lower limbs. What is the most likely underlying diagnosis?

- [ ] **A** Addison's disease
- [ ] **B** Diabetes mellitus
- [ ] **C** Grave's disease
- [ ] **D** Tuberculosis
- [ ] **E** Ulcerative colitis

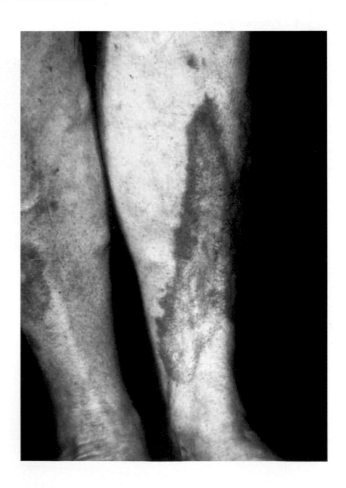

Answer on p. 44

33. This patient has been receiving a number of different treatments in hospital over the past 3 weeks. Which one of the following medications is most likely to have caused this adverse effect?

☐ **A** Aciclovir

☐ **B** Co-amoxiclav

☐ **C** Co-trimoxazole

☐ **D** Penicillin

☐ **E** Ritonavir

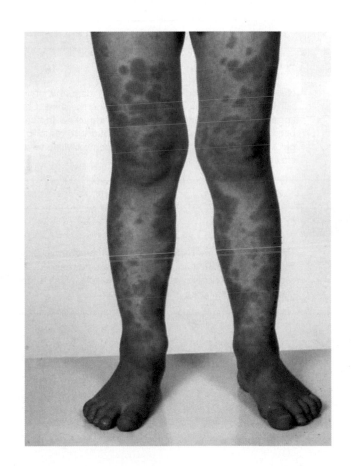

Answer on p. 44

31. **D: Pyoderma gangrenosum**

The classic ulcerative form is very painful and begins as a nodule or sterile pustule progressing to a necrotic and purulent ulcer, with an oedematous, blue-black expanding border (part a). The aetiology is unknown, and around two-thirds of cases are associated with other disease, including inflammatory bowel disease, seropositive or seronegative arthritides, multiple myeloma, paraproteinaemia, and leukaemia. Other extra-gastrointestinal features of Crohn's disease are uveitis, spondylarthropathy and primary sclerosing cholangitis.

32. **B: Diabetes mellitus**

Necrobiosis lipoidica (diabeticorum) is an idiopathic granulomatous skin disorder that typically occurs overlying the shins. Characteristic appearance is an erythematous patch with yellowish hue that becomes progressively atrophic. It is thought to respond to better glycaemic control; corticosteroids and pentoxifylline have been effective in some cases.

33. **C: Co-trimoxazole**

The appearances are typical of erythema multiforme. Drugs most commonly implicated are allopurinol, carbamazepine, cephalosporins, ciprofloxacin, co-trimoxazole, NSAIDs, penicillins, rifampicin, sulfasalazine and vancomycin.

34. A 24-year-old man presents with a 4-week history of lower back pain and stiffness associated with dysuria. Which one of the following organisms is most likely to be associated with development of this condition?

    A *Candida albicans*

    B *Chlamydia trachomatis*

    C *E. coli*

    D Herpes simplex

    E *Salmonella typhi*

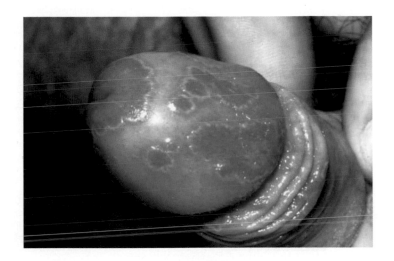

Answer on p. 48

35. This 43-year-old woman presents with a 5-day history of intermittent fever symptoms. On examination, there is a soft systolic murmur, and a rash overlying her trunk. Which one of the following is the most likely explanation for her rash?

- A Discoid lupus erythematosus
- B Discoid psoriasis
- C Erythema chronicum migrans
- D Erythema marginatum
- E Erythema multiforme

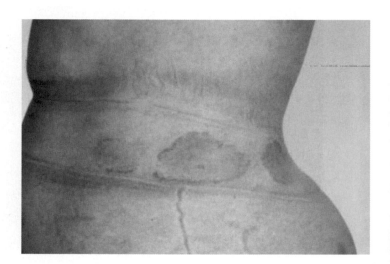

Answer on p. 48

36. A 32-year-old woman presents with abdominal pain and nausea, and is found to have a serum sodium concentration of 132 mmol/l. Which is the most likely underlying diagnosis?

- A Addison's disease
- B Hypothyroidism
- C Polyarteritis nodosa
- D Vitiligo
- E Wegener's granulomatosis

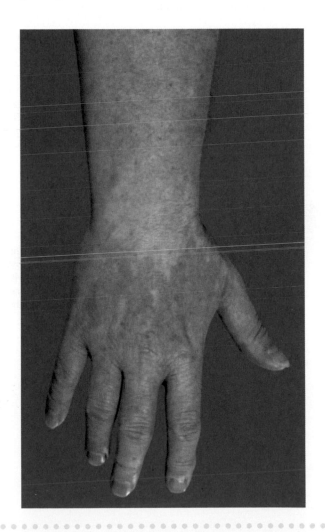

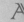

34. **B: *Chlamydia trachomatis***

Reiter's disease is one of a group of 'reactive' arthritides, and is a post-infective inflammatory disorder that most commonly occurs after infection with *Salmonella*, *Shigella*, *Chlamydia trachomatis* and *Ureaplasma urealyticum*.

35. **D: Erythema marginatum**

Rheumatic fever is an inflammatory disorder that is a delayed sequel to group A streptococcal pharyngitis, and is still a major cause of heart disease in the developing world. Major clinical manifestations include carditis, migratory polyarthritis, chorea, erythema marginatum (transient pink rash with raised margin, present in 20% of cases) and subcutaneous nodules. It can manifest as an acute fever, migratory polyarthritis, carditis and Sydenham's chorea. Penicillin is the most appropriate primary and secondary prophylaxis. Anti-inflammatory agents provide symptomatic relief but do not prevent rheumatic heart disease.

36. **A: Addison's disease**

Vitiligo is an asymptomatic autoimmune disorder involving destruction of melanocytes and depigmentation. It is associated with a number of other autoimmune disorders. Treatment with topical immunomodulators (eg tacrolimus and pimecrolimus) can help in some cases, and micropigment injection (tattooing) may be helpful.

37. A 33-year-old woman had recently been diagnosed with irritable bowel syndrome by her GP. She now presents with an intensely itchy rash. What is the most likely underlying diagnosis?

A Coeliac disease

B Contact dermatitis

C Crohn's disease

D Guttate psoriasis

E HIV infection

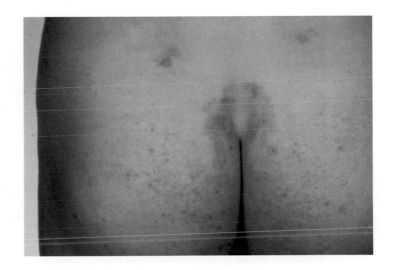

38. This 61-year-old man has been treated in hospital for recurrent generalised seizures and suspected pneumonia. He has developed a fever, has a reduced conscious level and an exfoliative rash. Which one of the following drugs is most likely to be responsible?

- A Carbamazepine
- B Ciprofloxacin
- C Erythromycin
- D Diazepam
- E Phenytoin

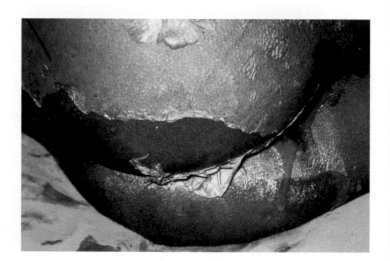

Answer on p. 52

39. A 58-year-old woman is rushed to the A&E department with sudden onset of severe central chest pain associated with palpitations. Taking the ECG appearances into account, which of the following coronary artery territories is most likely to be involved?

- [ ] **A** Anterior circumflex artery
- [ ] **B** Left anterior descending artery
- [ ] **C** Marginal artery
- [ ] **D** Posterior circumflex artery
- [ ] **E** Right coronary artery

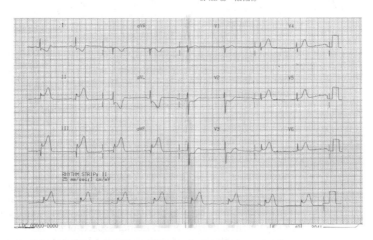

21 MAR 05   16:13:18

37. A: Coeliac disease

The vesicular appearance suggests dermatitis herpetiformis, an intensely itchy vesicular rash that is caused by IgA deposition in the papillary dermis; all have gluten-sensitive enteropathy, even if asymptomatic. The diagnosis of coeliac disease is often difficult, and many patients describe vague symptoms such as fatigue and mild gastrointestinal disturbance, which can easily be misinterpreted as irritable bowel syndrome.

38. A: Carbamazepine

Toxic epidermal necrolysis gives appearance similar to second-degree burn injuries, and results from drug metabolites toxic to keratinocytes. Mortality rate is 25–30% due to secondary sepsis and metabolic derangement. Corticosteroid treatment may worsen prognosis. Other recognised causes of fatal toxic epidermal necrolysis include lansoprazole, NSAIDs, penicillins and sulfonamides.

39. E: Right coronary artery

The ECG shows ST segment elevation consistent with acute inferior myocardial infarction (MI). Coronary anatomy is variable, but the right coronary artery (and its lesser branches) typically supplies the SA and AV nodes, inferior and posterior aspects of the left ventricle and the right ventricle. Bradyarrhythmia is a frequent complication after inferior MI.

40. A 58-year-old woman presents with a short history of weight loss and fatigue, and is found to have a rash overlying her trunk and abdomen. What is the most likely underlying diagnosis?

- [ ] **A** Breast carcinoma
- [ ] **B** Cutaneous T-cell lymphoma
- [ ] **C** Ovarian carcinoma
- [ ] **D** Pancreatic carcinoma
- [ ] **E** Strongyloides infestation

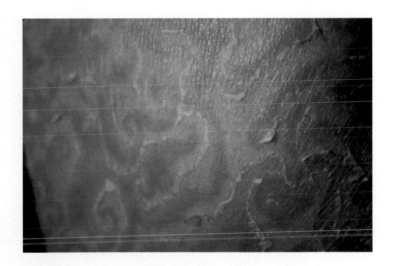

41. A 29-year-old Afro-Caribbean man attends the outpatient clinic for investigation of a painful genital ulcer. What is the most likely explanation for the appearance shown?

    ☐ **A** Behçet's disease

    ☐ **B** Chancroid

    ☐ **C** Genital herpes

    ☐ **D** Squamous carcinoma

    ☐ **E** Syphilis

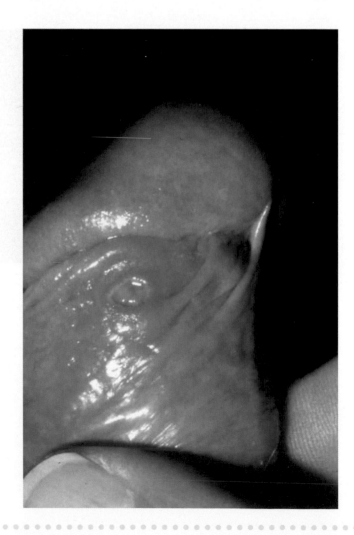

Answer on p. 56

42. This 54-year-old man presents to the general medical outpatient clinic for investigation of fatigue and leg cramps. On examination, resting heart rate is 54 beats per minute, blood pressure 146/82 mmHg and the jugular venous waveform is elevated to the angle of the jaw. What is the most likely explanation for the skin changes in his legs?

- A Chronic heart failure
- B Cutaneous T-cell lymphoma
- C Grave's disease
- D Hashimoto's thyroiditis
- E Hypothyroidism

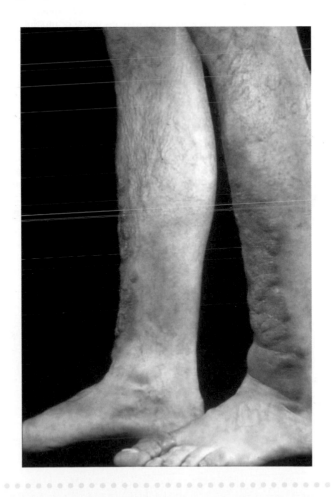

40.   A: Breast carcinoma

Erythema gyratum repens is associated with underlying breast and lung carcinoma. Typically, the rash is transient and moves around, and has well defined concentric rings. Necrolytic migratory erythema is associated with underlying glucagonoma, and has a less well circumscribed appearance.

41.   B: Chancroid

Caused by *Haemophilus ducreyi* and is the commonest cause of genital ulceration worldwide; may be single or multiple ulcers. Syphilitic chancre may give a similar appearance but is characteristically painless. Ulcers of chancroid tend to be deeper than those of herpes and bleed more easily.

42.   C: Grave's disease

Pretibial myxoedema is an autoimmune disorder, characteristically associated with Grave's disease, but can also occur in patients with Hashimoto's thyroiditis. Almost all cases have some degree of ophthalmopathy and high titres of anti-thyroid-stimulating hormone receptor antibody. The disorder is independent of clinical thyroid status.

43. This patient presented with a painless foot ulcer. What is the most likely underlying diagnosis?

☐ **A** Arterial embolisation

☐ **B** Diabetes mellitus

☐ **C** Homocystinuria

☐ **D** Varicose veins

☐ **E** Vasculitis

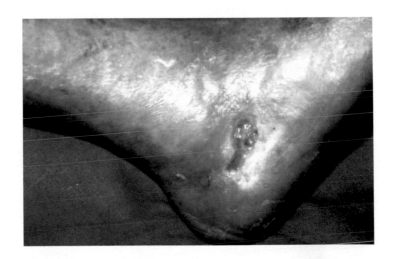

44. A 32-year-old schoolteacher is referred to hospital for investigation of cough, fever and general malaise over the past 6 days. Plain chest radiograph is shown below. Which infectious organism is most likely to be responsible for the abnormality shown?

A *Bacteroides* spp.

B *Haemophilus influenzae*

C *Legionella pneumoniae*

D *Mycoplasma pneumoniae*

E *Streptococcus pneumoniae*

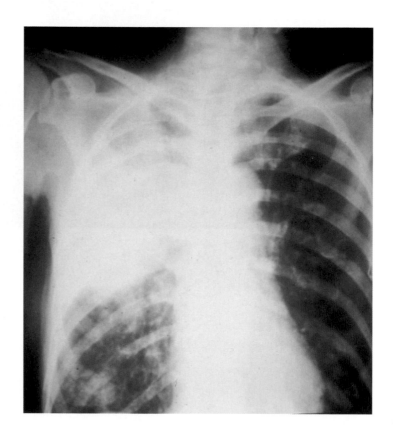

Answer on p. 60

45. A 35-year-old male bartender presents with mild fever and a dry cough over the past week. His peripheral oxygen saturation is 98% at rest but falls to 92% during clinical examination at the bedside. What infectious organism is most likely to account for the abnormalities shown on his plain chest radiograph?

A *Aspergillus fumigatus*

B *Klebsiella pneumoniae*

C *Mycobacterium tuberculosis*

D *Pneumocystis carinii*

E *Pseudomonas aeruginosa*

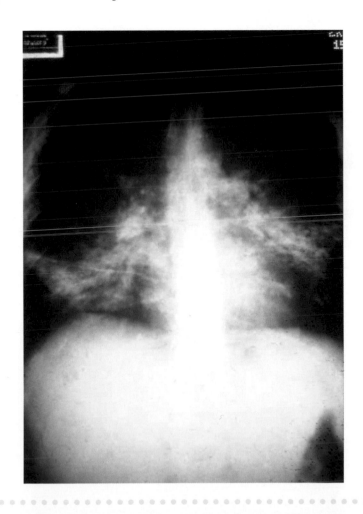

Answer on p. 60

43. **B: Diabetes mellitus**

Cumulative lifetime incidence of foot ulcers is around 15% in patients with diabetes mellitus. Sensorimotor neuropathy leads to increased pressures at foot surfaces, which may predispose to foot ulcers. Usually, these are painless, at sites of contact pressure and may have a deep punched out appearance. Other less common causes include syphilis, vitamin B_{12} deficiency, and chronic alcohol excess.

44. **E:** *Streptococcus pneumoniae*

This organism accounts for the majority of cases of community-acquired pneumonia. Other recognised but less common causes include *Chlamydia pneumoniae, Haemophilus influenzae, Legionella pneumoniae, Mycoplasma pneumoniae* and the influenza virus.

45. **D:** *Pneumocystis carinii*

The comparative lack of clinical features despite very extensive consolidation changes seen on the chest radiograph is suggestive of *Pneumocystis carinii* pneumonia, and haemoglobin desaturation on minimal exertion is a characteristic feature.

46. A 66-year-old lifelong smoker presents with breathlessness and haemoptysis. His chest radiograph is shown below. Which of the following features might most strongly suggest a Pancoast tumour?

A Anhidrosis affecting the right side of the face

B Excess salivation

C Left-sided facial droop

D Miosis of the left eye

E Mydriasis of the left eye

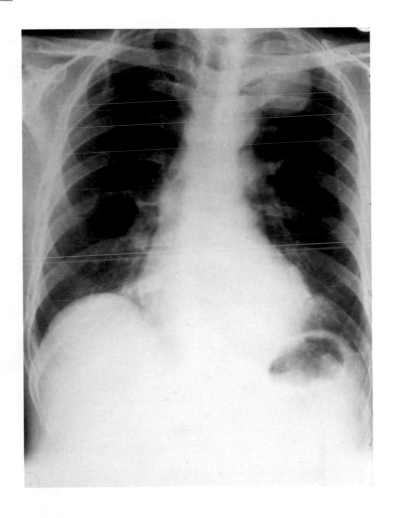

47. A 33-year-old male smoker presents with sudden onset of chest pain and breathlessness. On examination, oxygen saturation is 97%, pulse rate is 102 beats per minute and respiratory rate 20 breaths per minute. Which one of the following diagnoses best explains the findings shown on his plain chest radiograph?

- **A** Acute asthma
- **B** Acute pulmonary embolisation
- **C** Hyperventilation syndrome
- **D** Panic attack
- **E** Pneumothorax

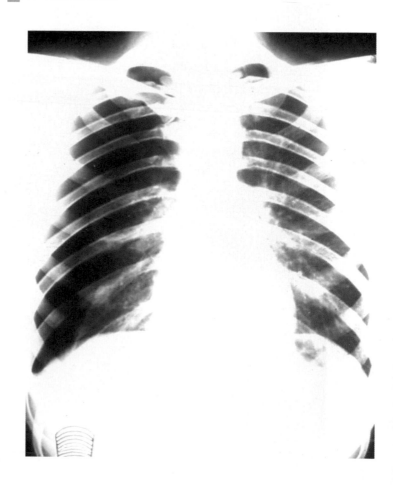

Answer on p. 64

48. A 67-year-old man presents with progressive breathlessness. His chest radiograph is shown. What two of the following diagnoses are most likely?

- [ ] **A** Asbestosis
- [ ] **B** Chronic obstructive pulmonary disease (COPD)
- [ ] **C** Coarctation of the aorta
- [ ] **D** Congestive heart failure
- [ ] **E** Mesothelioma
- [ ] **F** Previous asbestos exposure
- [ ] **G** Previous tuberculosis disease

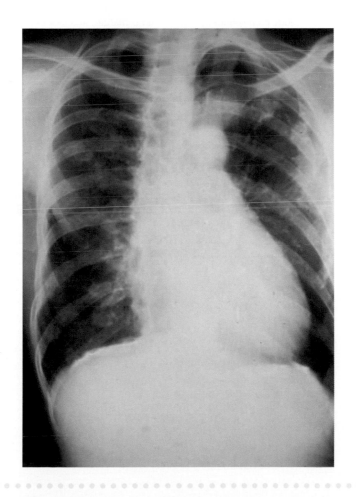

46. **D: Miosis of the left eye**

Pancoast tumour is an apical lung tumour with local neural plexus infiltration that results in ipsilateral Horner's syndrome (miosis, anhidrosis, partial ptosis) and wasting of the small muscles of the hand (T1 nerve root involvement).

47. **E: Pneumothorax**

Tension pneumothorax with partial collapse of the right lung is seen. There is relative over-inflation of the right hemi-thorax, a visible linear edge corresponding with the lung margin, and lack of any peripheral lung tissue markings beyond.

48. **B: Chronic obstructive pulmonary disease (COPD), F: Previous asbestos exposure**

Pleural plaques are seen in the pleura overlying the left lung field and diaphragmatic lung surfaces, which are indicative of previous asbestos exposure. The lung fields are hyperinflated, consistent with COPD but there are no specific features to indicate asbestosis (fibrosis). There is cardiomegaly, which might suggest an underlying diagnosis of hypertension or chronic heart failure, although there are no other features in support of the latter diagnosis.

49. This 38-year-old man had previously been well, and presented with a 6-week history of dry cough associated with a rash overlying both shins. Chest radiograph is shown below. What treatment is indicated on the basis of these findings?

A Combined rifampicin and isoniazid for 3 months

B Cyclophosphamide therapy for 4 months

C High dose corticosteroids for 6 months

D Observation only

E Sulfasalazine treatment for 4 months

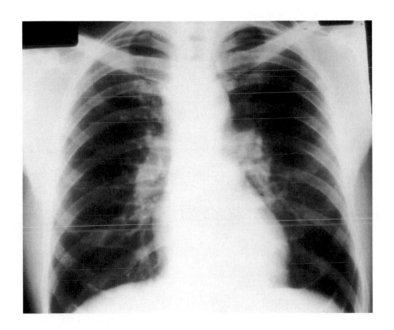

50. Which two of the following conditions are most likely to be responsible for development of the features seen in this chest radiograph?

- A Congestive heart failure
- B Cystic fibrosis
- C Miliary TB infection
- D *Pneumocystis carinii* pneumonia
- E Previous measles infections
- F Recurrent pulmonary embolus
- G Varicella pneumonia

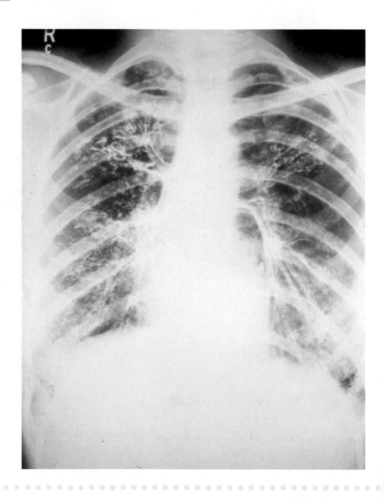

Answer on p. 68

51. This 48-year-old man presented to the A&E department with recurrent headaches. What is the most likely diagnosis?

A Basal skull fracture

B Meningioma

C Paget's disease

D Prolactinoma

E Sickle cell disease

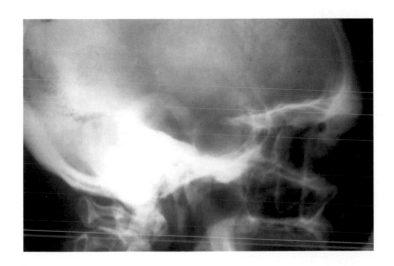

49. **D: Observation only**

Bilateral hilar lymphadenopathy without pulmonary infiltration indicates stage I sarcoidosis (stage II: hilar lymphadenopathy and lung infiltration, stage III: lung infiltration without hilar adenopathy). Stage I sarcoidosis rarely requires treatment, unless symptomatic relief is required for very painful erythema nodosum.

50. **B: Cystic fibrosis, E: Previous measles infections**

The bronchogram shows typical features of bronchiectasis. Other recognised causes are mechanical (tumour, foreign body), post-infective, TB, sarcoidosis, hypogammaglobulinaemia and ciliary dyskinesia.

51. **D: Prolactinoma**

There is gross expansion of the pituitary fossa, suggesting a large, progressively growing pituitary tumour.

52. Which of the following diagnoses is most likely to explain the abnormal appearances seen in this plain skull x-ray investigation in a 63-year-old man?

◻ **A** Beta-thalassaemia

◻ **B** Metastatic prostatic carcinoma

◻ **C** Multiple myeloma

◻ **D** Paget's disease

◻ **E** Sickle cell disease

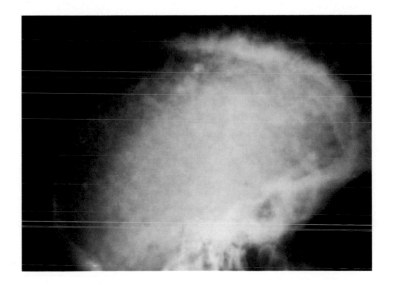

53. A 76-year-old man is admitted to the acute medical admissions unit for investigation of recurrent falls associated with transient loss of consciousness. Which two abnormalities are seen in the ECG?

A 2:1 atrioventricular block

B Atrial fibrillation

C Atrial flutter

D Complete heart block

E Rightward axis deviation

F Sinus arrhythmia

G Supraventricular tachycardia

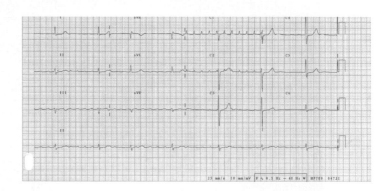

Answer on p. 72

54. This 54-year-old woman has been complaining of back pain for the past 2 months. What underlying diagnosis is most likely to account for the abnormalities shown on plain x-ray of the thoracolumbar spine?

- A Alkaptonuria
- B Ankylosing spondylitis
- C Chronic renal failure
- D Hypoparathyroidism
- E Metastatic breast cancer

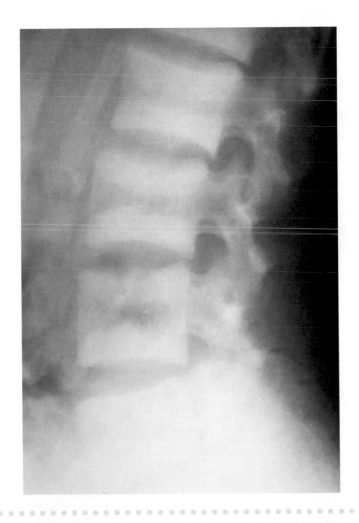

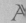

52. **D: Paget's disease**

Paget's bone disease affects around 5% of adults over 60 years of age, and is usually diagnosed on the basis of radiographic features. The skull shows marked cortical thickening with osteoporosis and osteosclerosis. Aetiology is unknown but several genetic loci have been identified from linkage studies.

53. **C: Atrial flutter, D: Complete heart block**

Flutter waves with characteristic saw tooth appearance are seen in V1 with rate around 150/min. The ventricular response is slow, and not associated with preceding atrial activity.

54. **C: Chronic renal failure**

There are band-like regions of increased opacity (sclerosis) at the superior and inferior margins of the vertebral bodies with intervening lucency, which gives rise to the classical appearance of 'rugger jersey' spine. This is virtually pathognomonic of secondary hyperparathyroidism of chronic renal failure, so-called renal osteodystrophy.

55. The following barium swallow investigation was performed on a 43-year-old man with a two-week history of progressive dysphagia. What is the most likely explanation for the appearances shown?

- [ ] **A** Achalasia
- [ ] **B** Candidiasis
- [ ] **C** Intra-mural T-cell lymphoma
- [ ] **D** Plummer–Vinson syndrome
- [ ] **E** Varices

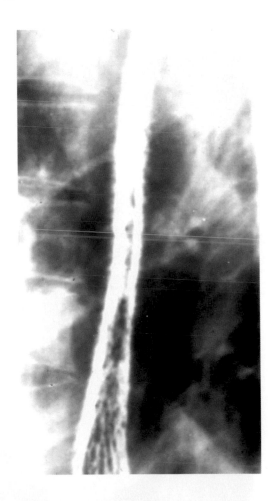

56. A 67-year-old woman has recently been treated with a number of courses of antibiotic therapy for cellulitis affecting the left lower limb. She has suffered intermittent abdominal pain and diarrhoea. What underlying cause of her gastrointestinal symptoms is indicated by this contrast enema study?

- A Diverticulitis
- B Pneumatosis coli
- C Pseudomembranous colitis
- D Small bowel obstruction
- E Ulcerative colitis

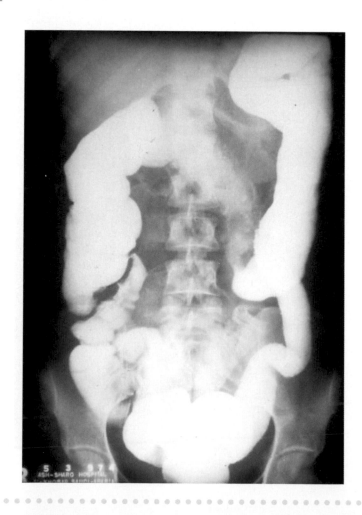

Answer on p. 76

57. A 73-year-old vagrant man is admitted via the A&E department having been found unresponsive in the street. He has a past history of alcohol abuse and generalised seizures. What is the most likely explanation for the abnormalities shown in the CT head scan?

- A Calcified haematomata
- B Cysticercosis
- C Intracerebral haemorrhage
- D Metastatic prostatic carcinoma
- E Tuberculomata

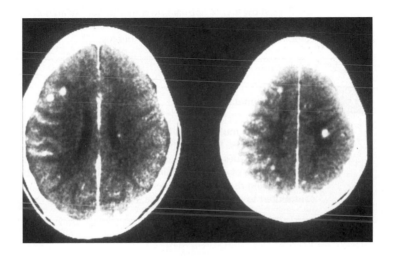

55. **B: Candidiasis**

Oesophageal candidiasis gives rise to an irregular 'shaggy' appearance to the mucosal surface. Extensive involvement indicates underlying impairment of T-cell-mediated immunity, for example AIDS or after cytotoxic chemotherapy.

56. **C: Pseudomembranous colitis**

The films show loss of normal bowel haustration, dilatation of large bowel and mucosal oedema. This is most likely to have arisen as a complication of prolonged antibiotic therapy.

57. **E: Tuberculomata**

These are often multiple, and have a predilection for the cerebral and cerebellar cortices. Mass lesions are approximately isodense with surrounding tissues, and seen more clearly in contrast studies due to an intense ring of contrast enhancement. Calcification may be present giving rise to a 'target sign'. Alcohol abuse is likely to have contributed to immunocompromise in this patient.

58. This 57-year-old patient is referred to the dermatology outpatient clinic for assessment. Which one of the following diagnoses is most likely to account for the abnormalities seen?

- [ ] **A** Digital embolisation
- [ ] **B** Malignant melanoma
- [ ] **C** Pyogenic granuloma
- [ ] **D** Subungual haematoma
- [ ] **E** Trauma

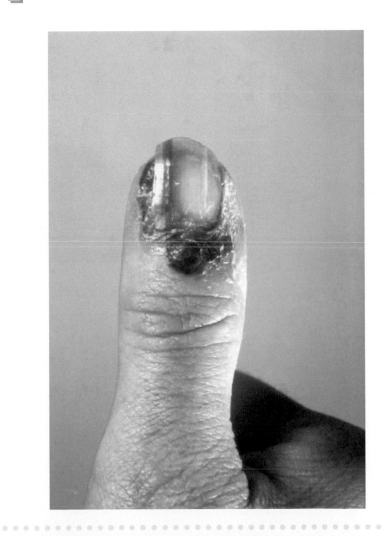

59. This 41-year-old woman presented to the A&E department with a painful left eye. Topical pilocarpine and fluorescein have been administered. What abnormality is shown?

- A Anterior uveitis
- B Corneal abrasion
- C Dendritic ulcer
- D Foreign body
- E Trachoma

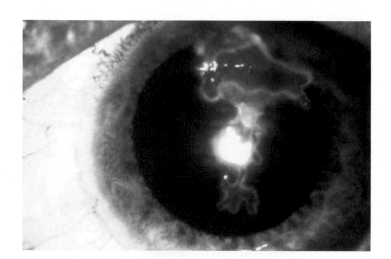

60. This 36-year-old man is noted to have multiple painless swellings around the neck. What is the most likely explanation for the appearances shown?

- ☐ **A** Branchial cysts
- ☐ **B** Carbuncles
- ☐ **C** Glandular fever
- ☐ **D** Multiple lipomata
- ☐ **E** Tuberculous lymphadenopathy

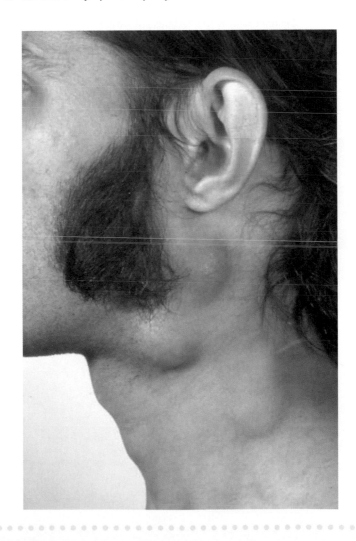

Answer on p. 80

58. | **B: Malignant melanoma**

Pigmented growth is seen throughout the nailbed. This is in contrast to the appearances of subungual haematoma, which is normally associated with proximal clearing with progressive nail growth.

59. | **C: Dendritic ulcer**

Dendritic ulcer is an infectious epithelial keratitis caused by herpes simplex virus, which characteristically involves superficial erosions with a branching morphological pattern. Herpes simplex can also cause stromal keratitis with deeper corneal involvement. Treatment is with topical aciclovir ointment; oral aciclovir may be used for prophylaxis in patients who develop multiple relapses.

60. | **E: Tuberculous lymphadenopathy**

Tuberculous lymphadenopathy is more common in immunosuppressed individuals. Painless multiple lymphadenopathy is often associated with Hodgkin's disease and non-Hodgkin's lymphoma. Glandular fever is a relatively common cause of cervical lymphadenopathy, but typically the glands are tender and it is usually accompanied by pharyngitis.

61. This 57-year-old lady is found to have protein +++ on dipstick urinalysis. What underlying disorder is suggested by her facial appearance?

- A Cushing's syndrome
- B Familial hypercholesterolaemia
- C Multiple myeloma
- D Nephrotic syndrome
- E Systemic amyloidosis

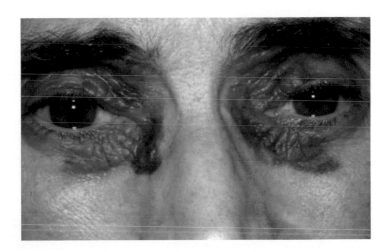

Answer on p. 84

62. This 52-year-old man is referred to the general medical outpatient department for investigation of progressive weight loss? What is the most likely explanation for the physical signs shown?

- [ ] **A** Grave's ophthalmopathy
- [ ] **B** Horner's syndrome
- [ ] **C** Myasthenia gravis
- [ ] **D** Myotonic dystrophy
- [ ] **E** Partial cranial nerve III abnormality

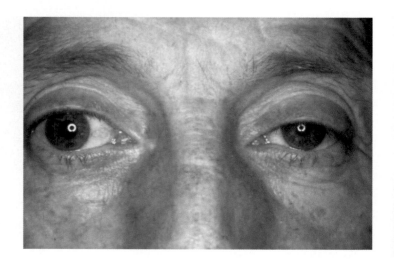

Answer on p. 84

63. This 68-year-old patient is referred to clinic for investigation following a number of simple falls at home. What is the most likely underlying diagnosis?

A Cushing's syndrome

B Grave's disease

C Horner's syndrome

D Myasthenia gravis

E Myotonic dystrophy

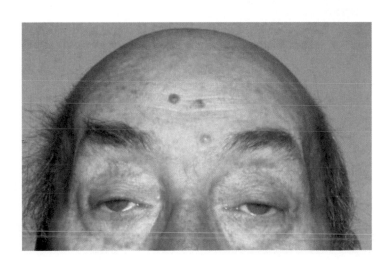

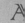

61. **E: Systemic amyloidosis**

Systemic amyloidosis with renal involvement is associated with heavy proteinuria, sometimes to nephrotic levels. There is often cardiac and gastrointestinal involvement, and small vessel fragility leads to easy bruising.

62. **B: Horner's syndrome**

Horner's syndrome results from disruption of the sympathetic nerve supply to the eye and face. Partial ptosis and meiosis are shown; other signs include ipsilateral anhidrosis around the eye and forehead. Potential causes include hypothalamic tumours, brainstem stroke, carotid artery injury and apical lung tumour. Rarely, it may be congenital.

63. **E: Myotonic dystrophy**

Myotonic dystrophy is characterised by bilateral partial ptosis, frontal baldness and failure of muscle relaxation after exercise. Myasthenia gravis is a recognised cause of bilateral partial ptosis, which is fatiguable, and typically found in younger female patients.

64. Which biochemical test would best establish the underlying diagnosis in this patient?

- ☐ **A** 24-hour urinary copper collection
- ☐ **B** Calcium and phosphate concentrations
- ☐ **C** Serum HDL and total cholesterol
- ☐ **D** Serum triglyceride
- ☐ **E** Total iron binding capacity

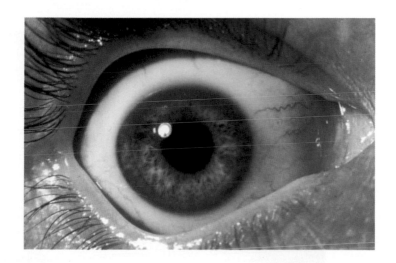

65. This 32-year-old patient has complained of intermittent headaches over the past 3 months. What is the most likely underlying diagnosis?

- [ ] A Benign intracranial hypertension
- [ ] B Grave's ophthalmopathy
- [ ] C Optic nerve Schwannoma
- [ ] D Phaeochromocytoma
- [ ] E Proliferative diabetic retinopathy

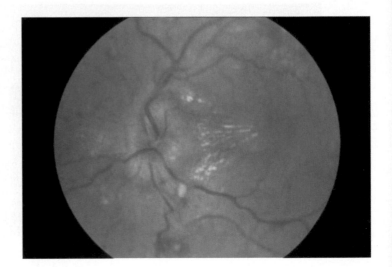

Answer on p. 88

66. This 64-year-old man is referred to the general medical outpatient department for investigation of progressive breathlessness over the past 6 weeks. What is the most likely explanation for the abnormalities shown on the plain chest radiograph?

- A Cardiac amyloidosis
- B Hypertrophic cardiomyopathy
- C Post-radiotherapy
- D Previous coronary artery bypass grafting
- E Previous tuberculosis infection

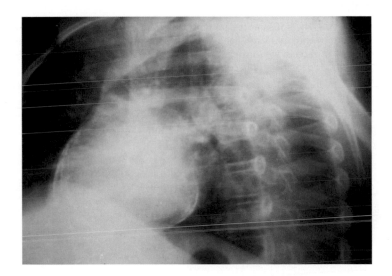

Answer on p. 88

64. **A: 24-hour urinary copper collection**

The appearances are those of Kayser-Fleischer, a brownish yellow ring in the outer cornea, which is pathognomonic for Wilson's disease. Diagnostic features include low serum caeruloplasmin, raised or normal total serum copper concentrations, and abnormally high serum non-caeruloplasmin-bound (free) copper.

65. **D: Phaeochromocytoma**

The appearances are typical of grade IV hypertensive retinopathy with exudates, haemorrhages and papilloedema. This indicates accelerated hypertension, which is associated with severe end-organ damage and necessitates prompt treatment.

66. **E: Previous tuberculosis infection**

A thin rim of calcification is seen corresponding with previous pericardial infection with tuberculosis. In this setting, the radiographic findings raise the possibility that constrictive pericarditis might account for breathlessness in this patient.

67. This 62-year-old woman is investigated for recent onset of visual disturbance. What is the most likely underlying diagnosis?

- **A** Atrial fibrillation
- **B** Hypercholesterolaemia
- **C** Multiple myeloma
- **D** Polyarteritis nodosa
- **E** Systemic lupus erythematosus

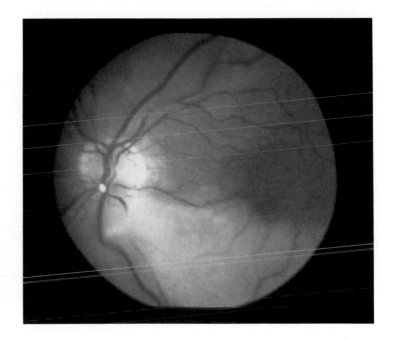

68. A 68-year-old man presents to the A&E department with central abdominal pain associated with nausea and vomiting. On examination, pulse rate is 88 beats per minute, supine blood pressure is 98/68 mmHg and sitting blood pressure 78/64 mmHg. What diagnostic test would be most useful in confirming the underlying diagnosis?

- **A** CT head scan
- **B** Serum amylase
- **C** Stool culture
- **D** Synacthen test
- **E** Urine osmolality

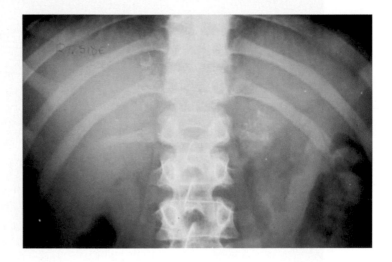

Answer on p. 92

69. A 56-year-old man is admitted with sudden onset of a painful, black second toe of the right foot. What is the most likely underlying diagnosis?

- **A** Cryoglobulinaemia
- **B** Erythroleukaemia
- **C** Multiple myeloma
- **D** Polycythaemia rubra vera
- **E** Sickle cell disease

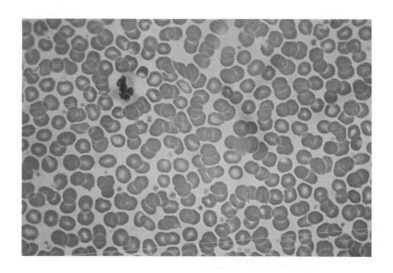

Answer on p. 92

67. **A: Atrial fibrillation**

The appearances indicate branch retinal artery occlusion (pallor and oedema). Characterised by painless sudden onset of unilateral visual field loss in the corresponding field, with afferent papillary defect. The mechanism is usually embolic (eg significant carotid atherosclerosis or atrial fibrillation), but may also be caused by inflammation (eg temporal arteritis) or suddenly increased intraocular pressure.

68. **D: Synacthen test**

The radiograph shows adrenal calcification, which is usually a consequence of previous tuberculous adrenalitis. The clinical features suggest hypoadrenalism, and the synacthen test would help confirm the diagnosis.

69. **D: Polycythaemia rubra vera**

PRV is a chronic myeloproliferative disorder where an abnormal clone gives rise to high circulating red cell concentrations, but may also be associated with high neutrophil and platelet concentrations. There is a significantly increased risk of venous and arterial thromboses. Hypochromic and microcytic cells may be seen due to co-existent iron deficiency anaemia.

70. A 34-year-old man presents with mild jaundice. What is the most likely explanation for his deranged liver biochemistry tests?

☐ **A** Coeliac disease

☐ **B** Hepatic vein thrombosis

☐ **C** Intra-hepatic artery occlusion

☐ **D** Intravascular haemolysis

☐ **E** Right ventricular dysfunction

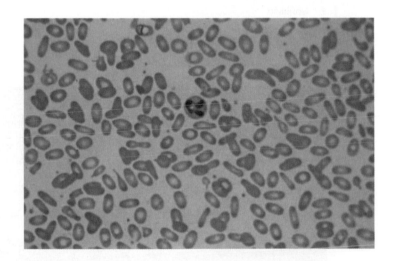

71. This peripheral blood film was taken from a 45-year-old woman who was undergoing hospital treatment of a febrile illness. Which two of the following treatments are most likely to account for the abnormal features shown?

- [ ] **A** Benzylpenicillin
- [ ] **B** Ciprofloxacin
- [ ] **C** Clarithromycin
- [ ] **D** Ibuprofen
- [ ] **E** Isoniazid
- [ ] **F** Paracetamol
- [ ] **G** Rifampicin

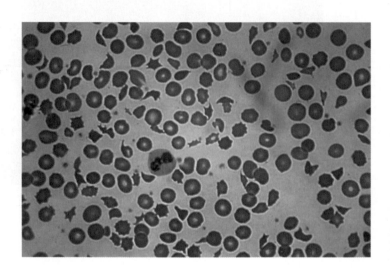

72. This peripheral blood film was from a 41-year-old man who was admitted to hospital for investigation of weight loss, fatigue and fever symptoms. What is the underlying diagnosis?

- [ ] **A** Acute myeloid leukaemia
- [ ] **B** Allergic pulmonary eosinophilia
- [ ] **C** Burkitt's lymphoma
- [ ] **D** Multiple myeloma
- [ ] **E** Waldenström's macroglobulinaemia

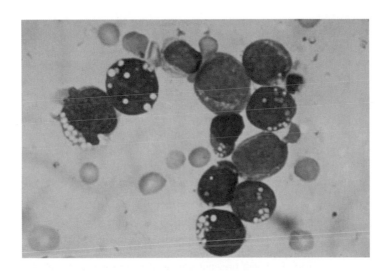

70. **D: Intravascular haemolysis**

Hereditary elliptocytosis is an uncommon disorder inherited in an autosomal dominant manner due to a defect of red cell membrane cytoskeleton. Most patients have normal haemoglobin concentrations, but evidence of compensated haemolysis. Extravascular haemolysis is more common than intravascular haemolysis. Complications include anaemia, jaundice and gallstones.

71. **A: Benzylpenicillin, B: Ciprofloxacin**

Schistocytes (fragmented red cells) and microspherocytes are features of haemolysis. Malarial parasites are not seen. Drug-induced autoimmune haemolysis is a recognised feature of penicillins, methyldopa, quinine and quinidine. In addition, patients with glucose-6-phosphate dehydrogenase deficiency are more susceptible to haemolysis, which may complicate treatment with quinolones, dapsone, aspirin, chloroquine and sulfonamides.

72. **C: Burkitt's lymphoma**

Burkitt's lymphoma frequently involves extranodal sites, with bone marrow and diffuse lymph node involvement. It is often seen in young adults and immune-compromised patients, and strongly associated with previous Epstein–Barr virus infection. Cells are of uniform size and shape, with scanty cytoplasm and round nucleus with slightly coarse chromatin and several nucleoli. There are frequent mitotic figures. The presence of a 'starry sky' appearance is given by scattered macrophages, and phagocytic debris is seen in Burkitt's lymphoma and other highly proliferative lymphomas.

73. What is the most likely underlying cause of the abnormalities seen in this 52-year-old man?

- [ ] **A** Charcot's arthropathy
- [ ] **B** Hypoparathyroidism
- [ ] **C** Psoriasis
- [ ] **D** Rheumatoid arthritis
- [ ] **E** Systemic lupus erythematosus

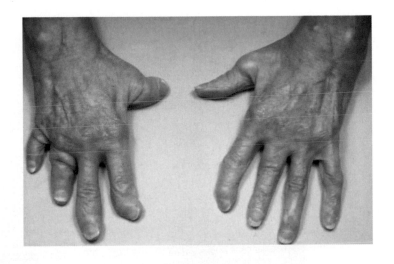

Answer on p. 100

74. This 58-year-old woman has longstanding type 1 diabetes mellitus. Which of the following would be most likely to prevent this complication?

  A Antihistamine administration

  B More frequent administration of smaller doses

  C Rotation of injection sites

  D Topical corticosteroid application

  E Use of recombinant human insulin

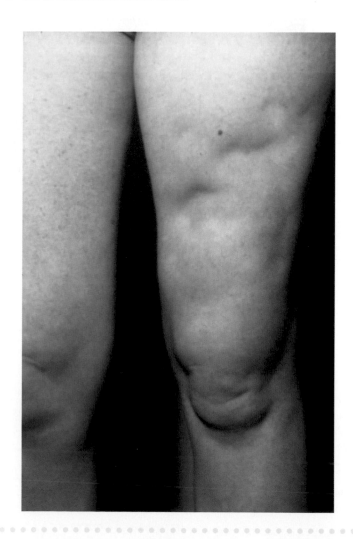

Answer on p. 100

75.   A 78-year-old woman presents to the A&E department with breathlessness. Which of the following diagnoses is most likely to account for the chest radiograph appearances?

☐ **A**   Dilated cardiomyopathy

☐ **B**   Mitral valve disease

☐ **C**   Pneumothorax

☐ **D**   Primary pulmonary hypertension

☐ **E**   Sarcoidosis

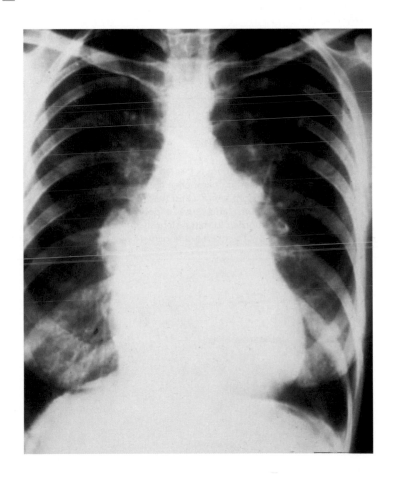

73. **C: Psoriasis**

Psoriatic arthropathy characteristically affects the distal interphalangeal joints. The appearances indicate telescoping of the ring and little fingers of the right hand, which is a feature of arthritis mutilans.

74. **E: Use of recombinant human insulin**

Lipoatrophy is an immunological reaction that does not occur with highly purified insulin types. Rotation of injection sites may reduce the cosmetic impact of lipodystrophies; corticosteroids and antihistamine treatments are of no benefit.

75. **B: Mitral valve disease**

The normal left atrium is located in the middle of the chest, and is the most posterior chamber of the heart. When it enlarges, it moves towards the right lateral chest wall (reaching it in patients with a giant left atrium), and causes a 'double bump' appearance to the right heart border. In mitral stenosis, the left atrial appendage may appear below the main pulmonary artery on the left heart border.

76. This is the barium meal investigation of a 56-year-old woman who has complained of longstanding intermittent dyspepsia. What is the diagnosis?

☐ **A** Gastric carcinoma

☐ **B** Gastric varices

☐ **C** Gastric outlet obstruction

☐ **D** Oesophageal stricture

☐ **E** Peptic ulceration

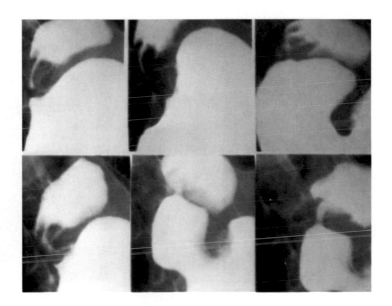

77. This 46-year-old woman is seen in the endocrinology outpatient clinic. You are asked to consider a possible diagnosis of Grave's disease. Which of the following features most strongly favours this?

A   Easy bruising

B   Lid lag

C   Tachycardia

D   Unilateral exophthalmos

E   Vitiligo

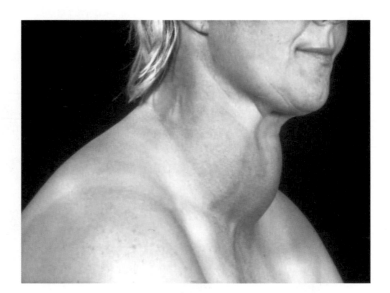

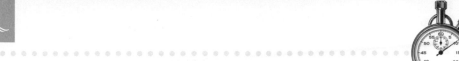

78. A 56-year-old man is admitted to hospital for investigation of nausea, vomiting, fever and right upper quadrant tenderness. What diagnosis is suggested by the appearances shown in his barium follow-through investigation?

  A Acute diverticulitis

  B Crohn's disease flare-up

  C Hepatic abscess

  D Small bowel obstruction

  E Small bowel perforation

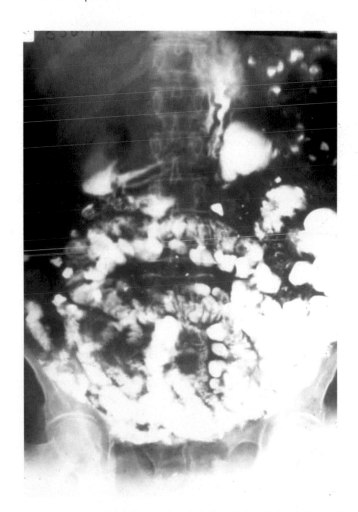

Answer on p. 104

76. **C: Gastric outlet obstruction**

In adults, pyloric stenosis is often secondary to scarring arising from recurrent peptic ulceration. This has become much less common because introduction of proton pump inhibitor therapy (eg omeprazole) has significantly improved the treatment of peptic ulcer disease.

77. **B: Lid lag**

Lid lag and tachycardia indicate hyperthyroid state, regardless of goitre. Specific features of Grave's disease are ophthalmopathy and pretibial myxoedema. Vitiligo is one of a number of autoimmune disorders that may be associated with Grave's disease.

78. **C: Hepatic abscess**

The appearances are of multiple diverticulosis affecting the small bowel. Recognised complications include acute diverticulitis, bacterial overgrowth, and bacterial seeding in the liver via the portal vein, which can result in hepatic abscess formation.

79. This 52-year-old lady was diagnosed with Raynaud's disease 4 years ago. She is referred to the medical outpatient department for investigation of progressively worsening breathlessness on exertion over the past 3 months. Which of the following antibody tests would be most helpful in establishing the underlying diagnosis?

- **A** Anticentromere
- **B** Anti-double-stranded DNA
- **C** Antinuclear antibody
- **D** Anti-Hu
- **E** Rheumatoid factor

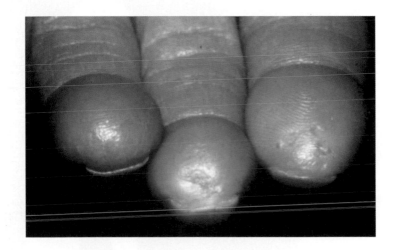

80. This barium enema was performed in a 34-year-old man who had complained of intermittent abdominal pain and altered bowel habit. What diagnosis is suggested by the abnormal appearance?

- **A** Collagenous colitis
- **B** Crohn's disease
- **C** Diverticular disease
- **D** Ischaemic colitis
- **E** Ulcerative colitis

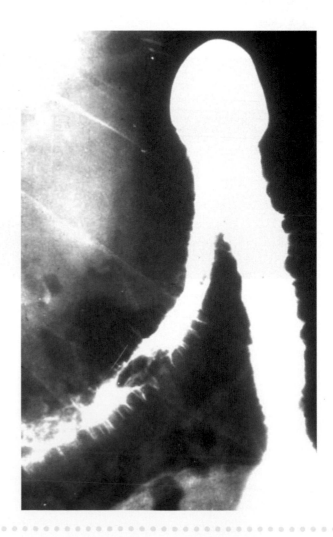

Answer on p. 108

81. This 56-year-old lady attended her GP complaining of a grating noise on mobilising her left knee. Which one of the following is the most likely underlying diagnosis?

- **A** Chondrocalcinosis
- **B** Diabetes mellitus
- **C** Haemophilia A
- **D** Pseudogout
- **E** Sarcoidosis

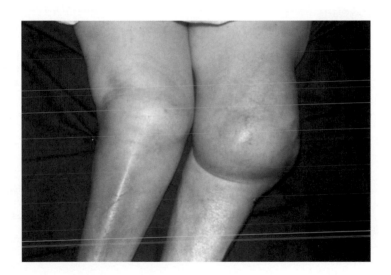

| 79. | A: Anticentromere |

Calcinosis seen affecting the fingertips, Raynaud's disease, oesophageal dysmotility, sclerodactyly and telangiectasia constitute CREST syndrome, in most of whom anticentromere antibody is positive. The clinical features suggest systemic sclerosis, in which anticentromere antibody is positive in 50–90%, and anti-SCL-70 antibody positive in 20–40%.

| 80. | B: Crohn's disease |

The enema demonstrates deep 'rose thorn' ulceration in the region of the transverse colon, which is a pathognomonic feature of Crohn's colitis. There is also evidence of mucosal oedema, suggesting acute disease activity.

| 81. | B: Diabetes mellitus |

This is a Charcot joint, characterised by painless joint destruction and deformity. It is seen in the setting of tertiary syphilis and other disorders that cause a sensory neuropathy (eg diabetes mellitus, amyloidosis and mixed sensorimotor neuropathy).

82. This 58-year-old man is referred to the cardiology outpatient department for investigation of chest pain. What underlying disorder is most likely to account for the abnormality seen on this plain chest radiograph?

☐ **A** Allergic bronchopulmonary aspergillosis

☐ **B** Hypertension

☐ **C** Myocardial infarction

☐ **D** Rheumatic fever

☐ **E** Tuberculosis

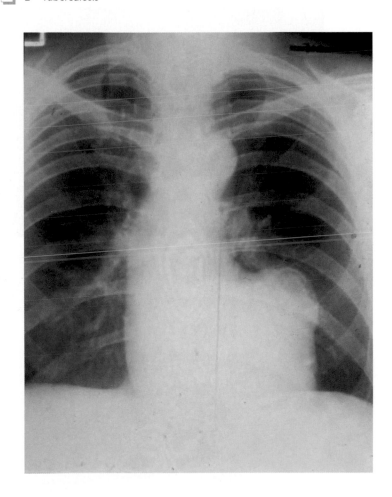

Answer on p. 112

83. This 55-year-old woman is found to have a painless pigmented lesion affecting the side of her neck. What is the diagnosis?

- A Discoid lupus erythematosus
- B Giant pigmented hairy naevus
- C Lentigo maligna
- D Nodular melanoma
- E Squamous cell carcinoma

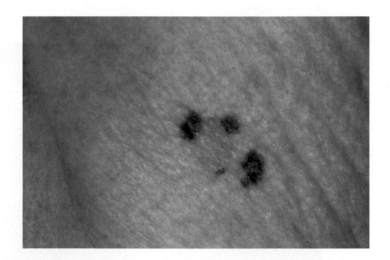

Answer on p. 112

84. This lateral skull x-ray film was taken from a patient with recurrent headaches. Which endocrine complication is most likely to be associated with this disorder?

- [ ] **A** Addison's disease
- [ ] **B** Cushing's syndrome
- [ ] **C** Diabetes insipidus
- [ ] **D** Diabetes mellitus
- [ ] **E** Phaeochromocytoma

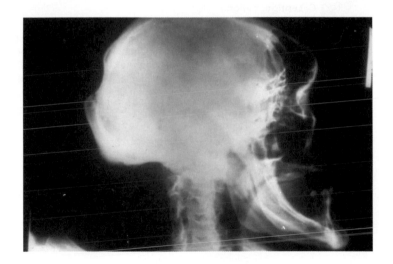

Answer on p. 112

82. C: Myocardial infarction

The radiograph shows the appearance of a left ventricular aneurysm, which is most commonly caused by previous transmural myocardial infarction. Recognised complications include thromboembolism, ventricular arrhythmia, congestive heart failure and cardiac tamponade.

83. C: Lentigo maligna

This disorder is characterised by flat pigmented lesions that expand slowly with central clearing of pigmentation. These typically occur in sun-exposed areas, typically affecting the cheeks of the face. This is an *in situ* variant of malignant melanoma, and development of raised papules is indicative of vertical invasion (lentigo maligna melanoma).

84. D: Diabetes mellitus

The skull x-ray appearances are those of acromegaly, with prognathism and frontal bossing. Diabetes mellitus is present in up to one-third of patients, and hypertension in up to 40%.

85. This 55-year-old man is assessed in the 'well man' clinic run at his GP practice. Which three of the following interventions would be expected to have greatest impact on delaying progression of this condition?

- ☐ **A** Antioxidant vitamin supplementation
- ☐ **B** Blood pressure-lowering therapy
- ☐ **C** Cholesterol-lowering therapy
- ☐ **D** Reduced dietary intake of refined carbohydrates
- ☐ **E** Regular aerobic exercise
- ☐ **F** Smoking cessation
- ☐ **G** Strict control of blood glucose concentrations
- ☐ **H** Weight loss

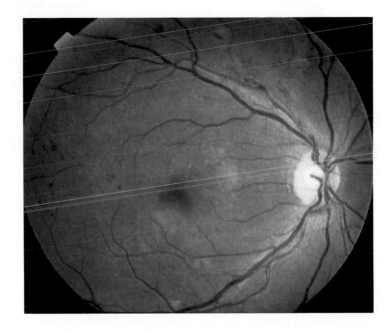

Answer on p. 116

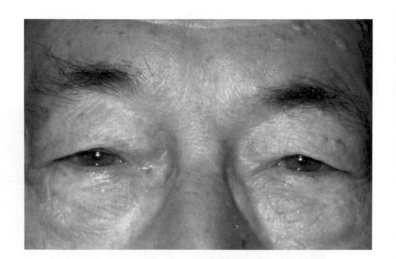

86. What test would be most helpful in establishing the underlying diagnosis in this 62-year-old woman?

A   24-hour urinary cortisol

B   Electromyography

C   Insulin stress test

D   Short synacthen test

E   Thyroid function tests

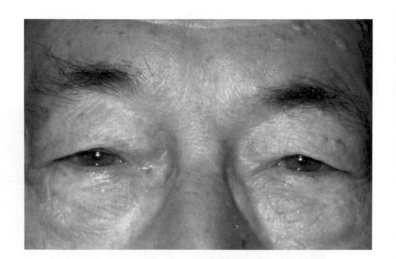

Answer on p. 116

87. A 34-year-old woman is referred to the general medical outpatient clinic for investigation of recurrent palpitations over the past 6 months. What is the most likely underlying diagnosis based on the appearance of her ECG?

A Caffeine excess

B Recurrent hypokalaemia

C Supraventricular tachycardia

D Tricyclic antidepressant toxicity

E Wolf–Parkinson–White syndrome

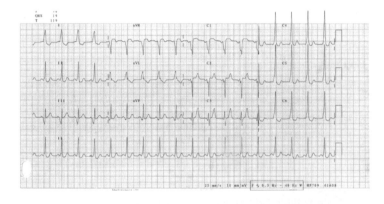

85. **B: Blood pressure-lowering therapy, C: Cholesterol-lowering therapy, G: Strict control of blood glucose concentrations**

Mild non-proliferative diabetic retinopathy. Tight control of blood glucose delays progression of microvascular complications of diabetes, and the benefits appear to be greatest if started early (eg primary prevention, before complications have occurred). Blood pressure lowering reduces the incidence of microvascular and macrovascular complications, and slows progression of retinopathy. High serum cholesterol concentrations are associated with increased retinal hard exudates, and high serum triglycerides increase the risk of proliferative diabetic retinopathy.

86. **E: Thyroid function tests**

Hypothyroidism is associated with dry coarse skin, pallor, hair loss (typically over the lateral third of the eyebrow), myopathy, obesity and dry brittle nails. Other features associated with hypothyroidism are slow-relaxing peripheral reflex responses, congestive heart failure and hypercholesterolaemia.

87. **E: Wolf–Parkinson–White syndrome**

Characteristic features are short PR interval <120 ms, due to conduction via aberrant pathway, followed by QRS with slurred upstroke (delta wave). Historically, it has been classified into a number of types including type A (predominantly positive QRS complexes in V1–V2) and type B (predominantly negative QRS complexes in V1–V2).

88. What is the most likely underlying diagnosis in this 54-year-old man?

- ☐ **A** Constrictive pericarditis
- ☐ **B** Hypothyroidism
- ☐ **C** Nephrotic syndrome
- ☐ **D** Superior vena cava occlusion
- ☐ **E** Wilson's disease

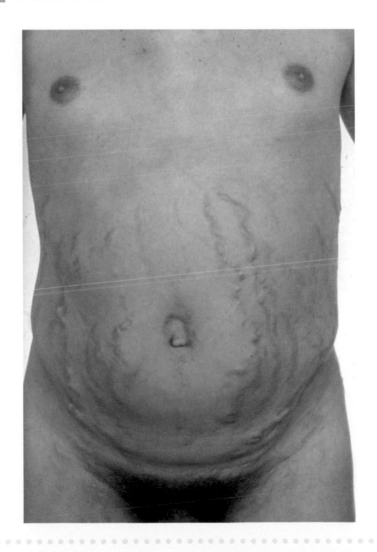

89. This 52-year-old man presented with progressive fatigue. Which of the following diagnoses best explains the abnormal clinical signs?

- **A** Alcoholic liver cirrhosis
- **B** Bronchogenic carcinoma
- **C** Congestive cardiac failure
- **D** Cushing's disease
- **E** Grave's disease

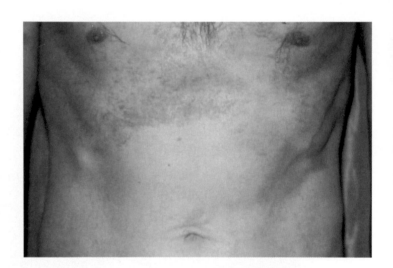

Answer on p. 120

90. This 46-year-old man presents with acute pain and redness overlying the first metatarsal joint of the left foot. Which two of the following drugs would be the most appropriate initial therapy?

☐ **A** Allopurinol

☐ **B** Benzylpenicillin

☐ **C** Codeine

☐ **D** Colchicine

☐ **E** Furosemide

☐ **F** Probenecid

☐ **G** Sulfasalazine

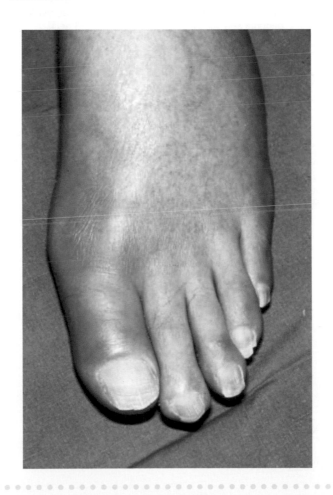

88.

E: Wilson's disease

Abdominal distension due to ascites, and dilated superficial abdominal veins due to portosystemic shunting, and gynaecomastia are recognised clinical features in liver cirrhosis.

89.

B: Bronchogenic carcinoma

Oedema and venous distension overlying the upper chest wall are recognised signs of superior vena caval obstruction. Recognised symptoms include sensation of fullness in head, blackouts and facial oedema and suffusion around the head and neck.

90.

C: Codeine, D: Colchicine

The appearance and site of the lesion are typical of acute gout. Immediate treatment is with colchicine, or a non-steroidal anti-inflammatory drug. Allopurinol may precipitate acute gout, and is introduced for prophylaxis only after the acute episode has resolved.

91. A 41-year-old woman with a 6-month history of crampy abdominal pain and intermittent diarrhoea undergoes a barium enema. What is the most likely underlying diagnosis?

- [ ] **A** Collagenous colitis
- [ ] **B** Crohn's colitis
- [ ] **C** Irritable bowel syndrome
- [ ] **D** Proctitis
- [ ] **E** Ulcerative colitis

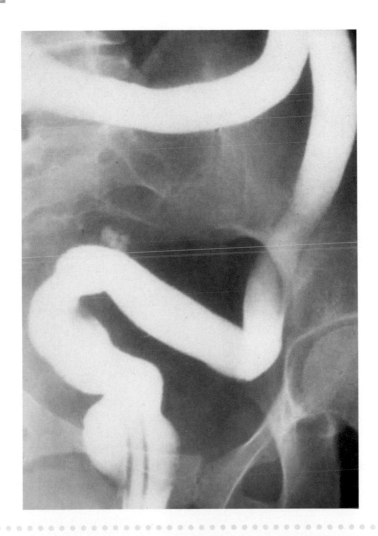

92. A 45-year-old man presents with progressive breathlessness on exertion. What initial investigation would be most helpful in establishing the underlying diagnosis?

- [ ] **A** Bronchoalveolar lavage
- [ ] **B** Chest wall ultrasonography
- [ ] **C** CT thorax
- [ ] **D** Sputum microscopy and Ziehl–Nielson staining
- [ ] **E** Pleural aspiration

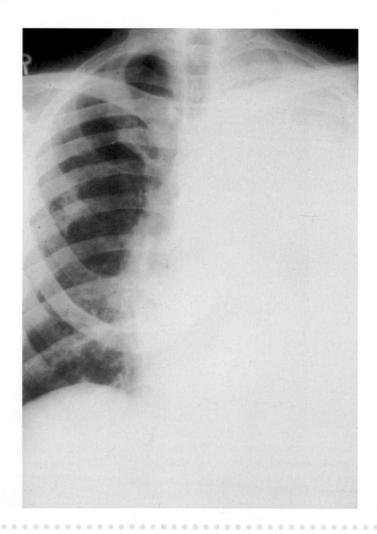

Answer on p. 124

93. This abdominal radiograph was performed in a 49-year-old man with a 6-month history of intermittent back pain. What is the most likely diagnosis?

- **A** Addison's disease
- **B** Chronic pancreatitis
- **C** Hydatid cyst disease
- **D** Renal tuberculosis
- **E** Ureteric calculus formation

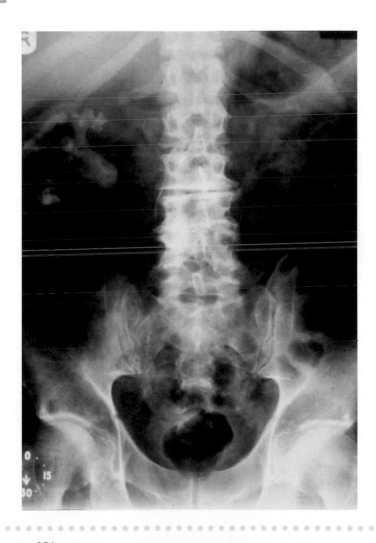

91.   **E: Ulcerative colitis**

The appearances are of chronic total panproctocolitis with a so-called leadpipe colon, which is a pathognomonic feature of ulcerative colitis. The colon is featureless, shortened, and haustrations are absent.

92.   **E: Pleural aspiration**

The chest radiograph shows a very large unilateral pleural effusion. Ultrasound scanning might be used to confirm the presence of fluid. Protein >30 g/l and lactate dehydrogenase >250 U/l are consistent with an exudate rather than a transudate. Aspiration with high neutrophil count might indicate empyema, which would require urgent treatment.

93.   **E: Ureteric calculus formation**

The plain radiograph shows calcification within the renal pelvis consistent with a staghorn calculus. The history of intermittent back pain might indicate obstructive uropathy, ureteric colic or superimposed pyelonephritis.

94. This 47-year-old patient presents to the A&E department with a painful and swollen left wrist. What diagnosis is indicated by the plain radiograph?

- [ ] **A** Metastatic thyroid carcinoma
- [ ] **B** Osteoblastoma
- [ ] **C** Osteomalacia
- [ ] **D** Paget's disease
- [ ] **E** Rickets

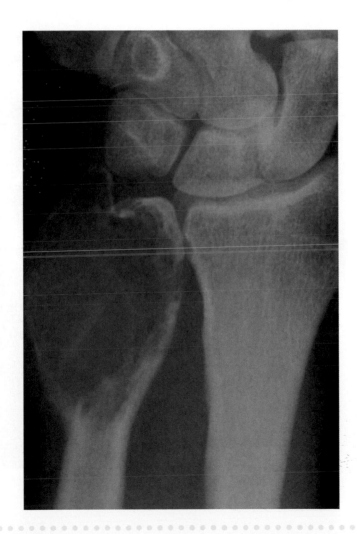

95. This 45-year-old man has longstanding inflammatory bowel disease. Over the past 4 days, he has suffered progressively worsening abdominal pain and fever symptoms. What complication has arisen?

- **A** Bowel perforation
- **B** Gastroparesis
- **C** Retroperitoneal fistula formation
- **D** Small bowel obstruction
- **E** Toxic megacolon

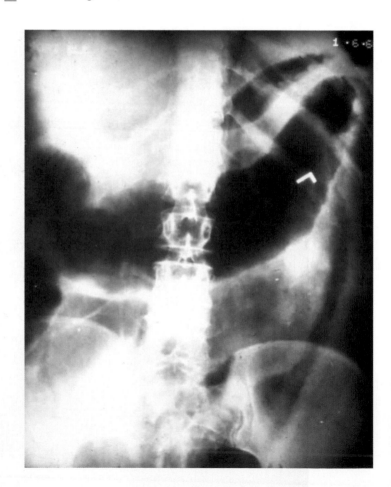

96. A 54-year-old man presents to the clinic with a short history of symptoms suggestive of Raynaud's phenomenon affecting both hands. What is the most likely underlying diagnosis?

- **A** Atrial fibrillation
- **B** Cryoglobulinaemia
- **C** Essential thrombocythaemia
- **D** Polycythaemia rubra vera
- **E** Systemic sclerosis

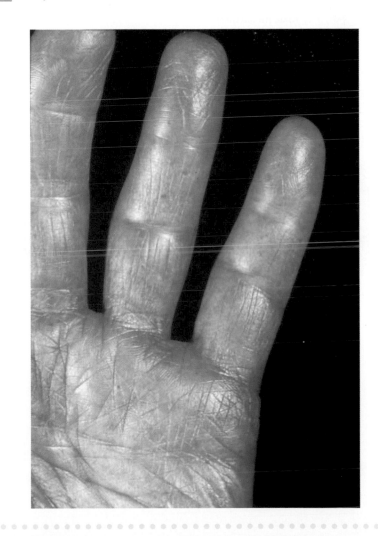

94.   **B: Osteoblastoma**

Osteoblastoma is an uncommon primary bone tumour that can result in debilitating pain. Recurrence after surgical resection is associated with more aggressive behaviour than the original tumour, therefore complete excision is important. Transformation to osteosarcoma is a recognised complication.

95.   **E: Toxic megacolon**

Toxic megacolon is a recognised severe complication of inflammatory bowel disease, pseudomembranous colitis and infectious gastroenteritis, for example caused by *E. coli*. Other potentially life-threatening complications of inflammatory bowel disease include thromboembolism, anterior uveitis and primary sclerosing cholangitis.

96.   **D: Polycythaemia rubra vera**

Raynaud's phenomenon is responsible for skin blanching in this patient. PRV is suggested by the erythematous appearance of both hands. PRV, cryoglobulinaemia and systemic sclerosis are recognised associations of Raynaud's phenomenon. Atrial fibrillation and essential thrombocythaemia may be associated with embolic digital infarction.

97. Contrast studies were performed in a 34-year-old man with a history of intermittent dyspepsia. What is the most likely diagnosis indicated by the appearance of the barium swallow?

☐ **A** Achalasia

☐ **B** Barrett's oesophagus

☐ **C** Cytomegalovirus oesophagitis

☐ **D** Oesophageal varices

☐ **E** Severe oesophageal candidiasis

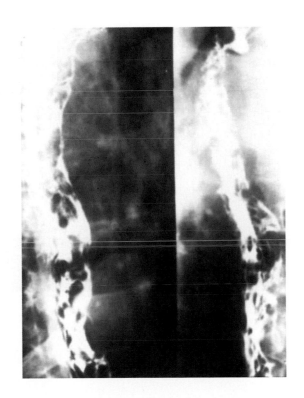

Answer on p. 132

98. This 48-year-old woman is complaining of pain and stiffness in her right hand. Which of the following is the most appropriate initial treatment?

A Allopurinol

B Co-amoxicillin

C Ibuprofen

D Prednisolone

E Sulfasalazine

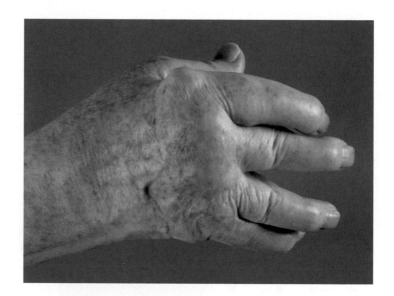

Answer on p. 132

99. This 58-year-old woman presented with a history of progressive weakness affecting her right upper limb. What underlying diagnosis is most likely to account for this appearance?

- ☐ **A** Amyloidosis
- ☐ **B** Compartment syndrome affecting the upper arm
- ☐ **C** Lead toxicity
- ☐ **D** Systemic lupus erythematosus
- ☐ **E** Thyrotoxicosis

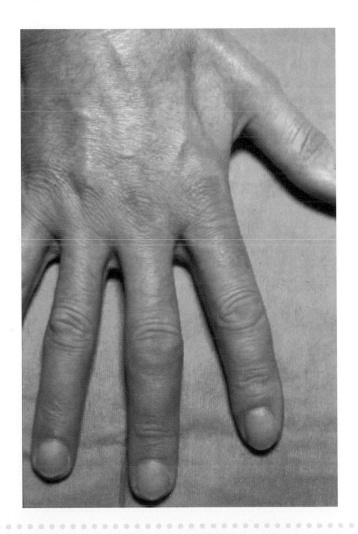

97. **D: Oesophageal varices**

Varices typically cause nodular, worm-like filling defects. These are distinct from the shaggy, irregular oesophageal mucosal outline seen in candidiasis.

98. **C: Ibuprofen**

The small joint deforming polyarthropathy is consistent with longstanding rheumatoid arthritis or gout. There is marked erythema, swelling and deformity of the metacarpophalangeal joints indicating an acute flare-up. NSAID treatment is appropriate initial management for analgesia, with consideration given to later treatment with disease-modifying drugs.

99. **D: Systemic lupus erythematosus**

There is muscle wasting of the first dorsal interosseous muscle, a distribution suggesting ulnar nerve palsy. Mononeuritis multiplex can also be caused by rheumatoid arthritis, neurofibromatosis, malignancy, sarcoidosis and (less commonly) amyloidosis. Lead toxicity can cause motor neuropathy, but this typically affects the lower limb.

100. This 46-year-old man is receiving treatment for Addison's disease and attends the endocrinology outpatient clinic for routine follow-up. He complains of blurred vision over the past 6–8 weeks. What is the most likely diagnosis?

- A Central serous retinitis
- B Papilloedema
- C Proliferative diabetic retinopathy
- D Retinoschisis
- E Retrobulbar lymphoma

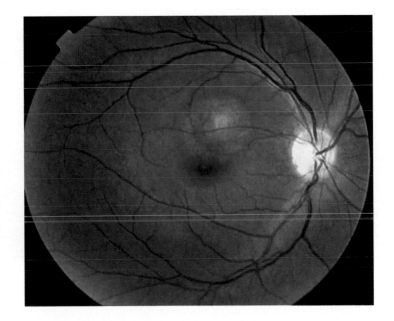

Answer on p. 136

101. This 64-year-old lady is under regular review in the general medical outpatient department, and normally wears glasses for reading. Four weeks ago, she noticed a sudden deterioration of her vision affecting her right eye. What is the most likely predisposing factor responsible for the appearances seen on fundoscopy?

- [ ] **A** Atrial fibrillation
- [ ] **B** Diabetes mellitus
- [ ] **C** Hypertension
- [ ] **D** Temporal arteritis
- [ ] **E** Waldenstrom's macroglobulinaemia

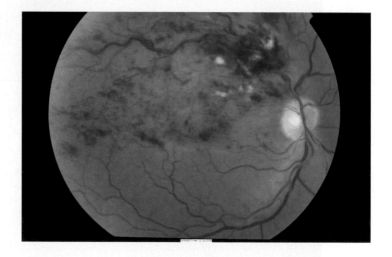

Answer on p. 136

102. A 56-year-old lady is referred to the DVT clinic by her GP for investigation of swelling in the region of the right popliteal fossa. An ultrasound scan with Doppler flow of the right popliteal fossa is shown below. What is the most likely diagnosis?

- ☐ **A** Arterio-venous malformation
- ☐ **B** Deep vein thrombosis
- ☐ **C** Femoral artery occlusion
- ☐ **D** Polyarteritis nodosa
- ☐ **E** Popliteal aneurysm

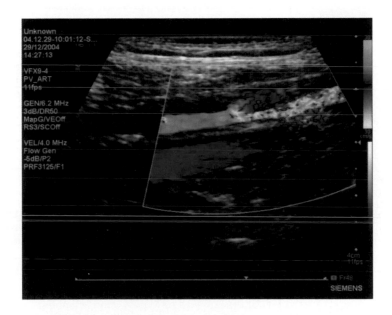

Answer on p. 136

100. A: Central serous retinitis

This is a relatively common retinal disorder, typically affecting young and middle-aged men. It is characterised by accumulation of subretinal fluid at the posterior pole of the fundus, creating a circumscribed area of serous retinal detachment. Risk factors are Cushing's syndrome, glucocorticoid treatment, stress and type-A personality traits, and pregnancy. Vision often recovers spontaneously within several months.

101. C: Hypertension

Branch retinal vein occlusion causes retinal vein dilatation, retinal haemorrhages and cotton-wool spots. It occurs in patients aged around 60 years, and the most common risk factors are hypertension (65%), diabetes mellitus (25%), valvular heart disease (25%) and carotid atheroma (45%). Rare causes include arteritis, vascular spasm and hyperviscosity syndromes.

102. E: Popliteal aneurysm

Popliteal artery shown superficial to the vein. There is laminar flow in the vein (shown in red). There is laminar flow in the proximal part of the popliteal artery (blue), a popliteal aneurysm associated with popliteal artery occlusion and turbulent flow distally.

103. This 49-year-old man had complained of breathlessness on exertion and fatigue. Routine blood tests show haemoglobin 9.7 g/dl and mean cell volume 116 fl. What is the most likely cause of his anaemia?

- A Azathioprine treatment
- B Homocysteinaemia
- C Hypothyroidism
- D Myelodysplasia
- E Vitamin B$_{12}$ deficiency

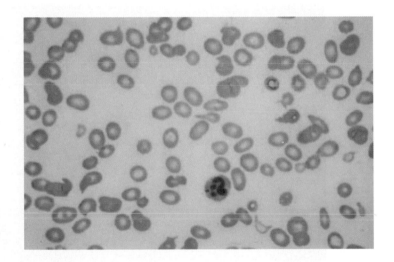

104. During a routine follow-up clinic appointment, this 36-year-old woman is noted to have a number of retinal abnormalities on fundoscopy. Which oral therapy would be most appropriate?

- [ ] **A** Aciclovir
- [ ] **B** Ganciclovir
- [ ] **C** Saquinavir
- [ ] **D** Valaciclovir
- [ ] **E** Valganciclovir

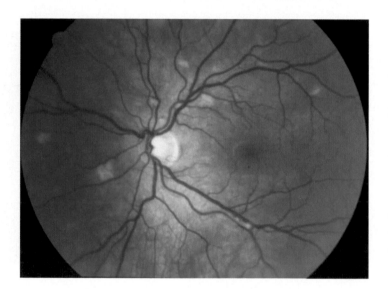

105. What is the most likely explanation for this rash, which is seen overlying the medial aspect of the foot?

- [ ] **A** Dermatitis herpetiformis
- [ ] **B** Erythema nodosum
- [ ] **C** Guttate psoriasis
- [ ] **D** Herpes zoster
- [ ] **E** Lichen planus

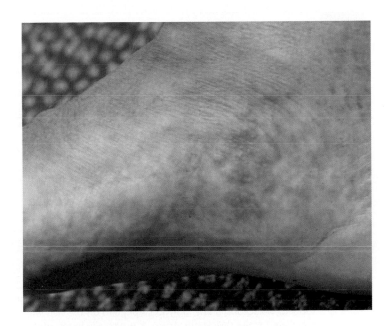

103. E: Vitamin B$_{12}$ deficiency

Hypersegmented neutrophils (>5 nuclear lobes) are an important diagnostic feature in the peripheral blood film, and indicate a disorder of neutrophil maturation. These are most commonly found in association with megaloblastic anaemia (vitamin B$_{12}$ and folate deficiencies) and in chronic diseases.

104. E: Valganciclovir

CMV remains the commonest cause of HIV-related retinitis, although its prevalence has fallen progressively since the introduction of highly effective anti-retroviral therapy. It is sight-threatening and is increasingly likely when CD4 count has fallen below 50/mm^3. Conditions other than HIV infection can predispose, for example lymphoma. Ganciclovir has greater activity than aciclovir (valaciclovir is a pro-drug of aciclovir), but is highly toxic. Valganciclovir is a pro-drug of ganciclovir with better oral absorption characteristics. Alternative treatments include foscarnet and cidofovir. Anti-CMV treatment can also be delivered by intravenous and intraocular routes.

105. E: Lichen planus

Lichen planus is a papulosquamous disorder involving skin and mucous membranes, nails and hair, and is characterised by flat-topped, violaceous, shiny, polygonal papules on the skin with thin reticulated scales (Wickham striae). It is typically found on the flexor surfaces of the upper extremities, genitalia, sacrum, lower extremities, scalp and nails. Atrophic cicatricial alopecia and nail fold destruction are recognised adverse effects. Oral lichen planus confers a 50-fold increased risk of oral cancer. Lichen planus is associated with the Koebner phenomenon.

106. This ECG was taken from a 74-year-old man who was referred to the medical outpatient department for investigation of recurrent falls associated with transient loss of consciousness, during which the patient is noted to look very pale. What of the following offers the most reasonable explanation for his falls?

☐ **A** Atrial fibrillation

☐ **B** Complete heart block

☐ **C** Sinus bradycardia

☐ **D** Supraventricular tachycardia

☐ **E** Ventricular tachycardia

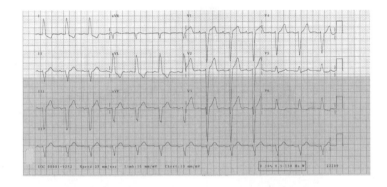

107. What is the most likely underlying explanation for this abnormal clinical sign in a 51-year-old asymptomatic man?

    A   Alcohol excess

    B   Chronic liver disease

    C   Epilepsy

    D   Idiopathic

    E   Repeated minor local trauma to hand

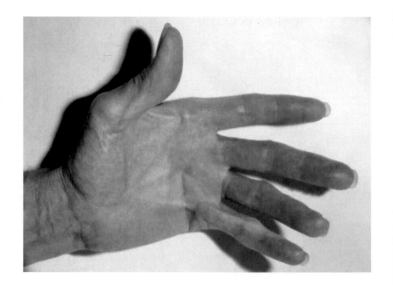

Answer on p. 144

108. This 56-year-old woman has longstanding rheumatoid arthritis. Which two of the following statements are correct with regard to the surgical procedure that has been undertaken?

- **A** Callosities resolve post-operatively
- **B** Deformity and pain are the main indications
- **C** Fusion arthroplasty is the preferred option in most cases
- **D** Long-term walking ability is improved in 90% of patients
- **E** Mal-alignment of the great toe is a frequent complication
- **F** Muscle strength improves post-operatively
- **G** Tendon laxity is a common adverse outcome

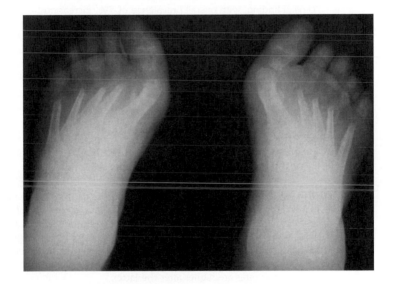

106. **B: Complete heart block**

The ECG shows tri-fascicular block, which is usually due to diffuse involvement of the cardiac conduction system by ischaemic heart disease. In this condition, comparatively small vagal stimuli or any further critical reduction in coronary blood flow can precipitate complete heart block.

107. **D: Idiopathic**

Dupuytren's disease (contracture not always present) is a common clinical finding, with overall prevalence of 4%, increasing to 20% in those aged over 65 years. There appears to be a genetic predilection, and it is more common in those of northern Europe descent. It becomes more common with age, and is more prevalent in those who drink alcohol excessively, and in patients with liver disease, diabetes mellitus and epilepsy, but these conditions are absent in the majority of cases.

108. **B: Deformity and pain are the main indications, E: Mal-alignment of the great toe is a frequent complication**

The patient has undergone bilateral excision of the metatarsal heads. Long-term outcome is poor due to forefoot pain, recurrence of the deformity and development of painful callosities. Recognised adverse effects are mal-alignment of the great toe, extensor tendon tightness and hindfoot deformity. Shoe fitting and correction of deformity are better than after fusion arthroplasty, and the complication and reoperation rates are higher after the latter.

109. This 56-year-old man was admitted with a 4-day history of fever and watery diarrhoea. A rash was noted overlying his upper and lower limbs. Which one of the following infective organisms is most likely to account for these features?

- **A** ECHO virus
- **B** Epstein–Barr virus
- **C** *Mycoplasma pneumoniae*
- **D** Rotavirus
- **E** Salmonella

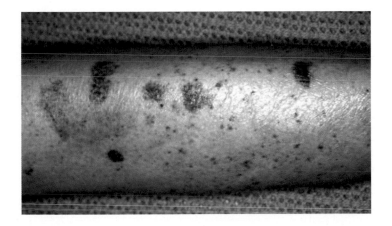

110. A 54-year-old woman is undergoing investigation of intermittent chest pain and palpitations. The electrocardiogram shown below was taken during stage 2 of a full Bruce protocol exercise test. What abnormality is shown?

☐ **A** Atrial fibrillation with aberrant conduction

☐ **B** Movement artefact

☐ **C** Ventricular fibrillation

☐ **D** Ventricular tachycardia

☐ **E** Wolf–Parkinson–White syndrome

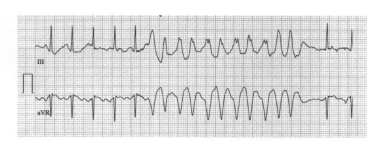

Answer on p. 148

111. The following pressure traces were obtained during cardiac catheterisation studies. During this 'pullback' study, the transducer is initially placed in the left ventricle and subsequently placed in the aorta. What diagnosis does this study most likely indicate?

A Aortic incompetence

B Aortic stenosis

C Left ventricular failure

D Mitral incompetence

E Ventricular septal defect

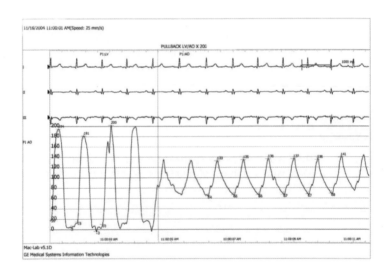

109. E: Salmonella

The prevalence of salmonella bacteraemia is 10-fold higher for non-typhii than *S. typhi* organisms. It is commonly associated with an erythematous rash or purpuric rash associated with underlying vasculitis. Ten per cent of patients with non-typhoidal Salmonella bacteraemia develop mycotic aneurysms.

110. D: Ventricular tachycardia

A self-limiting run of ventricular tachycardia may be a feature of underlying myocardial ischaemia. Significant myocardial ischaemia during an early phase of the Bruce exercise protocol warrants further investigation, and coronary arteriography should be considered.

111. B: Aortic stenosis

There is a significant pressure drop between the left ventricle and the aorta, with a gradient of more than 60 mmHg indicating severe stenosis.

112. This 64-year-old man is referred to the general medical outpatient department for investigation of progressive breathlessness on exertion. Which two of the following complications are most likely to account for breathlessness in this patient?

- [ ] **A** Amyloidosis
- [ ] **B** Cardiac failure
- [ ] **C** Kyphoscoliosis
- [ ] **D** Lung fibrosis
- [ ] **E** Metastatic lung disease
- [ ] **F** Pulmonary thromboembolism
- [ ] **G** Rib fracture

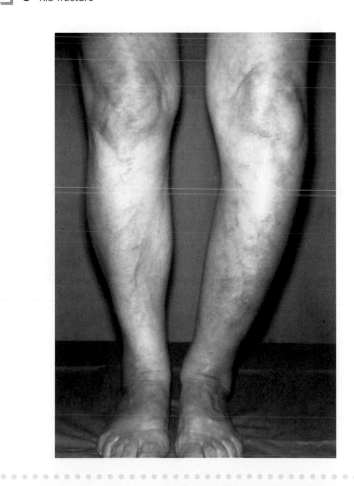

113. This 58-year-old woman presented with a 5-month history of headaches and intermittent fever symptoms. What is the most likely underlying diagnosis?

- [ ] **A** Histiocytosis X
- [ ] **B** Hyperparathyroidism
- [ ] **C** Metastatic breast carcinoma
- [ ] **D** Multiple myeloma
- [ ] **E** Paget's disease

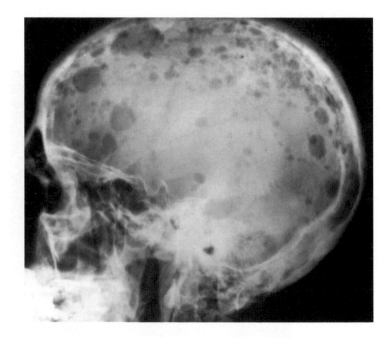

114. This 58-year-old patient is undergoing inpatient investigations to establish the cause of progressive breathlessness on exertion. Taking into account the appearance of the plain chest radiograph, what is the most likely diagnosis?

- ☐ **A** Congestive heart failure
- ☐ **B** Meig's syndrome
- ☐ **C** Pancreatitis
- ☐ **D** Recurrent pulmonary embolism
- ☐ **E** Tuberculosis

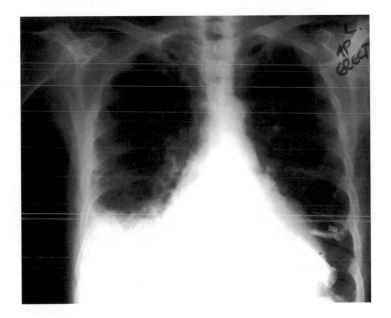

Answer on p. 152

112. **B: Cardiac failure, C: Kyphoscoliosis**

Tibia valga is consistent with Paget's disease. The plain x-ray film would be expected to show curved tibial margins with thickened cortices, and a technetium 99m bone scan would be expected to demonstrate increased isotope uptake.

113. **D: Multiple myeloma**

The plain x-ray film shows numerous discrete areas of radiolucency, with appearances typical of multiple myeloma. Diagnosis is established by demonstration of monoclonal gammopathy with immunoparesis and detection of urinary Bence-Jones protein. Other characteristic features are raised serum calcium concentration, high erythrocyte sedimentation rate and lytic lesions in long bones and axial skeleton.

114. **A: Congestive heart failure**

Pleural effusion with cardiomegaly is due to congestive heart failure in the vast majority of patients in routine practice. In 40% of cases, pleural effusions are unilateral, and the prevalence of right-sided effusions is twofold higher than for left-sided effusions. Acute pancreatitis is associated with effusion in 10–15% of cases. Meig's syndrome is the rare association of ascites, right-sided pleural effusion and ovarian fibroma.

152   Answers to Questions 112–114

115. This patient presented to the A&E department with pain and swelling affecting the lateral aspect of the right hand. What underlying diagnosis is indicated by this plain x-ray?

- **A** Myeloma
- **B** Osteomyelitis
- **C** Paget's disease
- **D** Pathological metacarpal fracture
- **E** Tuberculosis

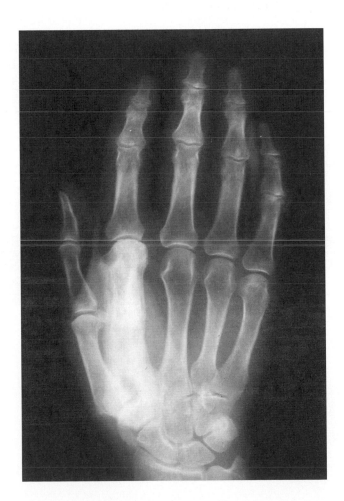

116. This 61-year-old man presented to the A&E department with progressive swelling and deformity affecting the right knee. What is the most likely explanation for the appearances shown on the plain knee x-ray?

☐ A Acute gout

☐ B Charcot's joint

☐ C Osteosarcoma

☐ D Severe rheumatoid arthritis

☐ E Tuberculous osteomyelitis

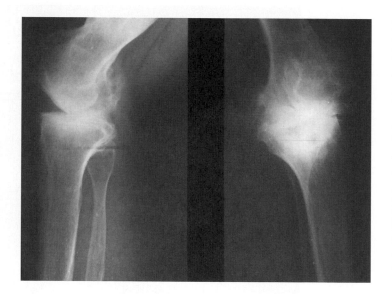

117. This 31-year-old woman has complained of intermittent pains in her hands and feet. What is the most likely underlying diagnosis?

- [ ] **A** Raynaud's disease
- [ ] **B** Reflex sympathetic dystrophy
- [ ] **C** Rheumatoid arthritis
- [ ] **D** Systemic lupus erythematosus
- [ ] **E** Systemic sclerosis

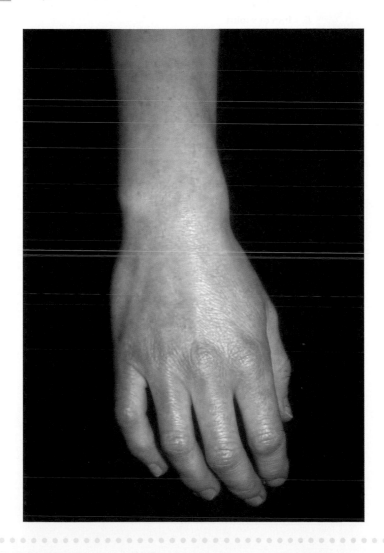

Answer on p. 156

115. **C: Paget's disease**

Paget's disease is characterised by irregular thickening of the cortices with increased opacification (osteosclerosis). These changes are seen affecting the first metacarpal. Close inspection is required to detect a possible pathological fracture at the site.

116. **B: Charcot's joint**

There is gross destruction of the knee joint, with obliteration of the normal joint space and peri-articular osteosclerosis. Charcot's joints were historically associated with neurosyphilis, but are now most commonly seen in patients with diabetes and sensory neuropathy.

117. **E: Systemic sclerosis**

Connective tissue disorder characterised by thickening and fibrosis of the skin (scleroderma), which looks tight and shiny, and fibrosis involving the gastrointestinal, renal and other organs. Three-quarters of patients have co-existent Raynaud's phenomenon.

118. This 58-year-old woman has longstanding chronic obstructive airways disease. Over the past three weeks, she has been receiving treatment for an exacerbation of her respiratory symptoms. A rash overlying her right arm developed four days ago. What is the most likely cause?

- A Erythema nodosum
- B Fixed drug eruption
- C Herpes zoster
- D Skin metastases from bronchogenic carcinoma
- E Tuberculosis infection

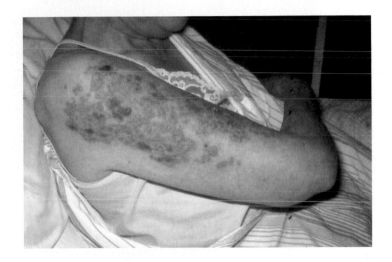

119. This 45-year-old man presented to the A&E department with a painful, red swelling overlying the left hand. Which one of the following antibiotic treatments is most likely to be effective?

- **A** Amoxicillin
- **B** Ciprofloxacin
- **C** Flucloxacillin
- **D** Tetracycline
- **E** Tinidazole

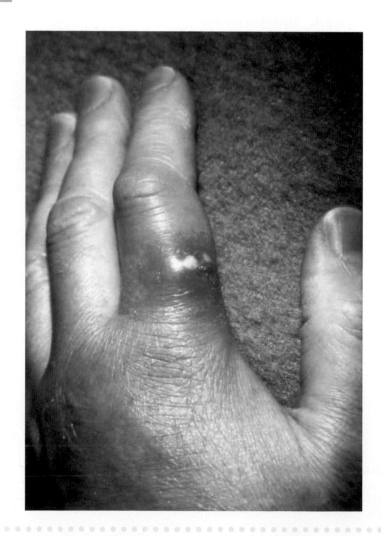

120. This 59-year-old woman is investigated for low back pain following a simple fall 3 days earlier. She is experiencing significant limitation of spine movement, with pain radiating towards the left iliac crest. Based on the appearance of the lateral lumbar spine x-ray, what is the most likely underlying cause?

A   Metastatic bone disease

B   Multiple myeloma

C   Osteomyelitis

D   Osteoporosis

E   Tuberculosis

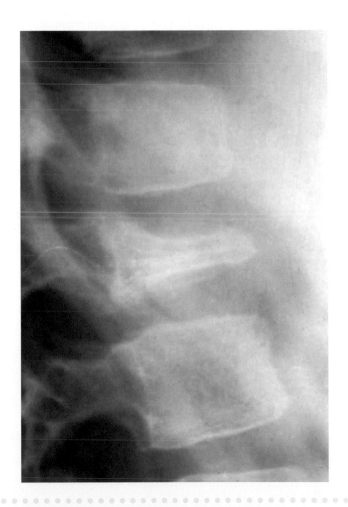

Answer on p. 160

118. **C: Herpes zoster**

The appearance is typical of herpes zoster, which is a recognised complication of immunosuppressive therapy (eg high dose corticosteroids). The site of the lesion suggests C7 dermatomal distribution.

119. **C: Flucloxacillin**

This patient has a carbuncle overlying the lateral aspect of the index finger, and the most commonly implicated organism is *Staphylococcus aureus*, which would be expected to be sensitive to flucloxacillin. Treatment should be guided by bacterial culture results and local sensitivities.

120. **D: Osteoporosis**

There is a wedge-shaped vertebral collapse, which is typically seen in trauma cases. The characteristic feature of osteoporotic vertebral collapse is reduction of vertebral bone density associated with widened inter-vertebral disc spaces.

121. This 33-year-old man has suffered progressive swelling and deformity. Which one of the following diagnoses is most likely to explain the abnormalities shown?

A Cholesterol embolisation

B Chronic tophaceous gout

C Lepromatous leprosy

D Neurofibromatosis

E Psoriatic arthropathy

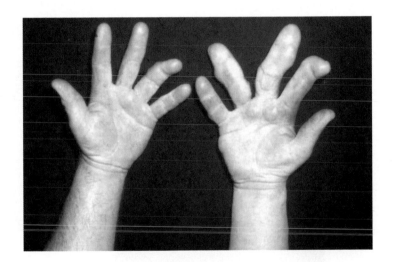

122. This 38-year-old man is referred to the general medical outpatient clinic for investigation of intermittent pain and paraesthesia of both hands. What is the most likely explanation for his symptoms?

    A Chondrocalcinosis

    B Hypocalcaemia

    C Median nerve compression

    D Osteomyelitis

    E Sensorimotor neuropathy

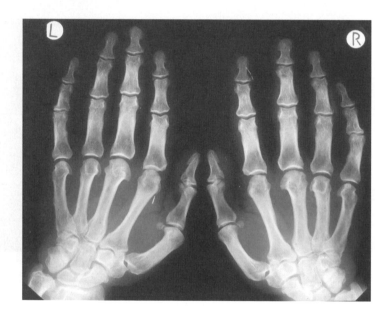

Answer on p. 164

123. This 38-year-old man is admitted for treatment of progressive breathlessness on exertion. He is found to have raised jugular venous pressure and cardiac auscultation reveals an added third heart sound. What is the most likely diagnosis?

A Diabetes mellitus

B Friedreich's ataxia

C Syringomyelia

D Systemic lupus erythematosus

E Thiamine deficiency

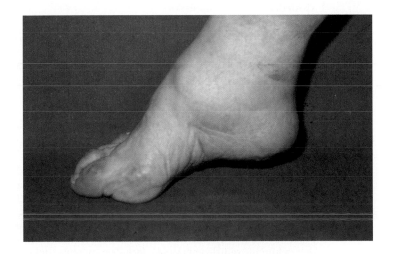

Answer on p. 164

121. **D: Neurofibromatosis**

Neurofibromatosis is associated with multiple neurofibromata, which may result in soft tissue swelling and organ infiltration. This patient had multiple neurofibromata causing soft tissue swelling and deformity of the hands. The patient underwent resection of a number of neurofibromata, and the diagnosis was confirmed histologically.

122. **C: Median nerve compression**

The plain x-ray appearances show elongation of the metacarpals and phalanges, in keeping with an underlying diagnosis of acromegaly. Recognised complications of acromegaly are carpal tunnel syndrome, diabetes mellitus and hypertension.

123. **B: Friedreich's ataxia**

There is no strict definition of pes cavus, but it is characteristically associated with a high arch that does not flatten on weight-bearing. Deformities associated with pes cavus include clawing of the toes, increased calcaneal angle, plantar fascia contracture as well as hyperextension of the great toe, and lead to metatarsalgia and callosities. Caused by a number of neuromuscular diseases (possibly due to intrinsic muscle imbalance), including muscular dystrophy, Charcot–Marie–Tooth disease, mononeuritis multiplex, polio, syringomyelia, Friedreich's ataxia and spinal cord compression. Friedreich's ataxia is often complicated by cardiomyopathy.

124. This 41-year-old woman is has been attending the hypertension clinic. Her most recent blood pressure recording is 156/104 mmHg despite taking atenolol 50 mg daily and nifedipine 30 mg daily. What diagnosis does this ^{131}I-meta-iodobenzylguanidine (MIBG) scintiscan indicate?

  ☐ **A** Chronic pyelonephritis

  ☐ **B** Conn's syndrome

  ☐ **C** Cushing's syndrome

  ☐ **D** Phaeochromocytoma

  ☐ **E** Renal artery stenosis

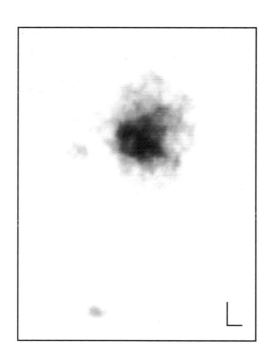

Answer on p. 168

125. A 27-year-old woman is admitted via the A&E department after deliberate overdose of amitriptyline 4 hours earlier. On the basis of the electrocardiogram appearance, which of the following treatments should most urgently be considered?

☐ **A** 10 ml 10% calcium carbonate intravenously

☐ **B** 100 mg intravenous atropine

☐ **C** 1.26% sodium bicarbonate infusion

☐ **D** Intravenous metoprolol

☐ **E** Oral verapamil

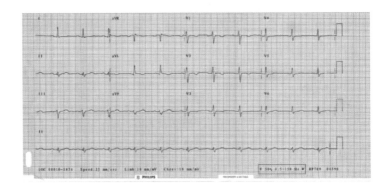

126. This 48-year-old man with severe hypertension recently underwent surgical intervention in an attempt to alleviate his high blood pressure. This biopsy specimen was excised during the operation. Which one of the following was most likely to have been responsible for his high blood pressure?

- A Acromegaly
- B Cushing's syndrome
- C Para-aortic lymph node compressing renal artery
- D Phaeochromocytoma
- E Wilm's tumour

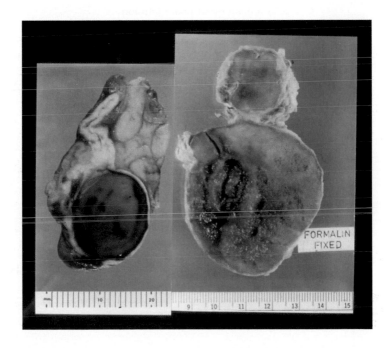

124. **D: Phaeochromocytoma**

The radioisotope ^{131}I-MIBG accumulates preferentially in these tumours of chromaffin tissue origin, in proportion to the extent of catecholamine synthesis. The scintiscan shows an area of high radionuclide uptake in the right supra-renal region, consistent with a unilateral functional (secretory) phaeochromocytoma arising from the adrenal medulla. Note that activity in the suprapubic region corresponds with normal urinary excretion of radiolabel.

125. **C: 1.26% sodium bicarbonate infusion**

There is minor prolongation of QRS duration (127 ms), which may be a toxic effect of tricyclic antidepressants in overdose, and indicates an increased risk of arrhythmia and seizures. Bicarbonate administration is thought to lessen the toxic effects of tricyclics on sodium channel activity, and may reduce arrhythmia and seizure risk. Note that the PR interval is also marginally increased, which is an uncommon feature.

126. **D: Phaeochromocytoma**

Typical waxy appearance on cross-section. The tumours are encapsulated or well-demarcated. The cut surface is variegated grey-tan to brown-red with areas of haemorrhage and cystic degeneration. The residual adrenal cortex is bright yellow. Resection allows restoration of normal blood pressure in some patients, but not all.

127. This 48-year-old man presented with chest pain at rest, associated with 2 mm ST segment depression in leads V4, V5 and V6. He undergoes urgent percutaneous transfemoral coronary arteriography with stent insertion in the left anterior descending coronary artery. What complication has most probably occurred?

☐ **A** Aspirin hypersensitivity

☐ **B** Cholesterol embolism

☐ **C** Femoral artery spasm

☐ **D** Thrombotic thrombocytopenic purpura

☐ **E** Warfarin-induced necrosis

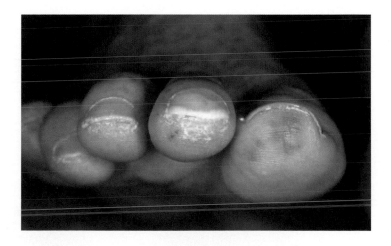

Answer on p. 172

128. This 48-year-old woman is referred to the acute medical admissions unit with rapidly progressive pain and swelling of her right foot over the past 2 days, associated with limitation of movement and fever symptoms. Investigations show haemoglobin 11.2 g/dl, white cell count 12.6 × 10⁹/l and serum urate 244 μmol/l. What is the most likely diagnosis?

- **A** Acute gout
- **B** Gonococcal arthritis
- **C** Psoriatic arthropathy
- **D** Pyrophosphate crystal deposition
- **E** Rheumatoid arthritis

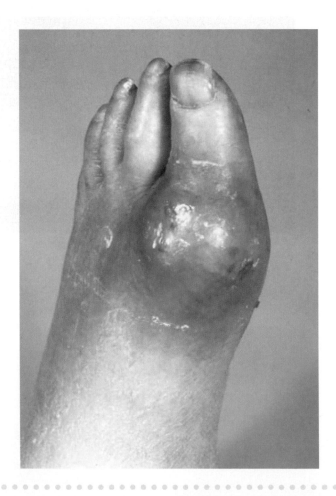

Answer on p. 172

129. This 56-year-old woman presented via the A&E department with two short-lived episodes of generalised seizure activity. Her partner reported that she had been suffering from right arm weakness over the past 6 weeks. What immediate therapy is most appropriate?

- [ ] **A** Cranial irradiation
- [ ] **B** Cytotoxic chemotherapy
- [ ] **C** Dexamethasone
- [ ] **D** Rifampicin
- [ ] **E** Vancomycin

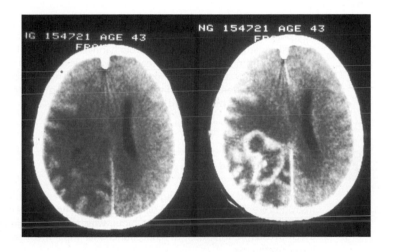

Answer on p. 172

127. **B: Cholesterol embolism**

Commonly occurs after invasive vascular access procedures, although may occur spontaneously. Can lead to 'trash' foot in more extensive cases. Other features of cholesterol embolism include fever, renal impairment and raised erythrocyte sedimentation rate and eosinophil count.

128. **A: Acute gout**

Psoriasis is complicated by arthropathy in a number of patterns: distal interphalangeal joint involvement, symmetrical deforming small joint polyarthropathy (resembling rheumatoid hands), asymmetric large joint monoarthritis (similar to osteoarthritis) and sacroiliitis, and arthritis mutilans. Gout is commonly associated with normal serum urate concentrations, although total body urate is often elevated, and urate crystals may be detected in synovial fluid.

129. **C: Dexamethasone**

This patient had a slow-growing glioblastoma, with a cystic and necrotic core. The CT head scan demonstrates significant oedema and inflammation surrounding the tumour, which can be minimised by corticosteroid treatment to reduce functional impairment and lower seizure risk.

130. These are the visual field charts for a 56-year-old man who presented with headaches and visual disturbance. Which two of the following disorders are most likely to account for the abnormality shown?

- ☐ **A** Acute glaucoma
- ☐ **B** Central retinal vein occlusion
- ☐ **C** Diabetic papillopathy
- ☐ **D** Grave's ophthalmopathy
- ☐ **E** Multiple sclerosis
- ☐ **F** Proliferative diabetic retinopathy
- ☐ **G** Pseudotumour cerebri

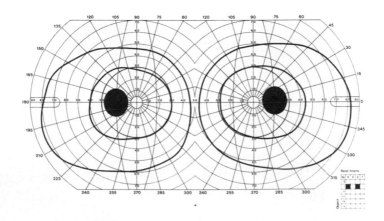

131. This 53-year-old man had been diagnosed with diabetes mellitus more than 25 years ago, and is under regular follow-up in the diabetes outpatient clinic. Which of the following statements is most likely correct regarding therapies used to treat the condition found during routine retinal screening?

- ☐ **A** Intravitreal ranibizumab reduces risk of cataract formation
- ☐ **B** Laser photocoagulation should not be undertaken in patients >50 years of age
- ☐ **C** Pan-retinal photocoagulation increases the risk of an early decrease in visual acuity
- ☐ **D** Photocoagulation confers less benefit in patients with type 2 diabetes
- ☐ **E** Scatter laser photocoagulation is reserved for highly advanced proliferative retinopathy

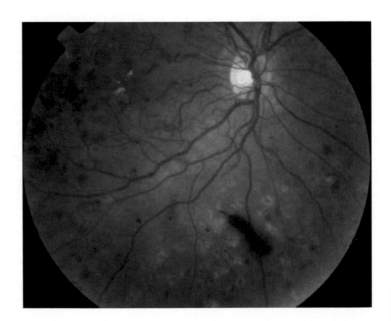

132. This 43-year-old man with long-standing type 1 diabetes mellitus presented via the A&E department with a 3-day history of abdominal pain and vomiting. What is the most likely explanation for his symptoms?

  A   Atonic colon

  B   Autonomic neuropathy

  C   Gastric outlet obstruction

  D   Gastroenteritis

  E   Small bowel obstruction

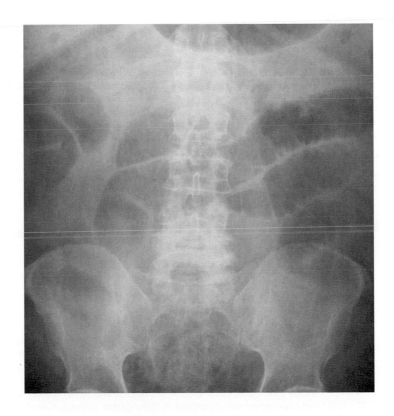

130. C: Diabetic papillopathy, G: Pseudotumour cerebri

The charts demonstrate blindspot enlargement, which is a feature of papilloedema and, in some cases, papillitis. Papilloedema can be associated with raised intracranial pressure (central venous thrombosis, tumour, abscess, benign intracranial hypertension), Cushing's syndrome, arachnoid cysts and intracranial arterio-venous anomalies. Acute idiopathic blind spot enlargement (AIBSE) is recognised in some patients without significant papilloedema.

131. C: Pan-retinal photocoagulation increases the risk of an early decrease in visual acuity

Proliferative diabetic retinopathy. Benefits of early pan-retinal photocoagulation laser treatment is greatest in those with type 2 diabetes older than 40 years with severe non-proliferative retinopathy or early proliferative retinopathy. Treatment can often be deferred in younger patients with type I diabetes. Complications include pain, visual-field loss, decreased dark adaptation, choroidal detachment and haemorrhage, tractional retinal detachment and choroidal neovascular membrane formation. Early macular oedema and visual acuity loss may occur; recovery is usually over 2–4 weeks but may be permanent. Pegaptanib (Eyetech Pharmaceuticals), ranibizumab (Genentech) and others are vascular epidermal growth factor (vEGF) inhibitors that have shown promising effects on maculopathy in early clinical trials. There is evidence of previous laser photocoagulation to the inferior and temporal regions.

132. E: Small bowel obstruction

Dilated loops of bowel can appear within hours of complete upper intestinal obstruction, or develop over longer periods where there is progressive small bowel obstruction. In long-standing obstruction, small bowel dilatation can mimic colonic dilatation. Distended small bowel loops tend to be seen in the central and upper abdomen, and valvulae coniventes distinguish it from gastric distension or dilated large intestine. Seventy-five per cent of cases are caused by adhesions; gallstone ileus is an unusual but recognised cause.

133. This 61-year-old woman was referred to the general medical outpatient department for investigation of intermittent abdominal pain and constipation over the past 6 months, associated with progressively worsening fatigue symptoms. Initial investigations show haemoglobin 9.6 g/dl and mean cell volume 71 fl. What is the most likely cause for these findings?

- [ ] **A** Caecal carcinoma
- [ ] **B** Chronic diverticulitis
- [ ] **C** Colonic abscess formation
- [ ] **D** Diverticular colitis
- [ ] **E** Ischaemic colitis

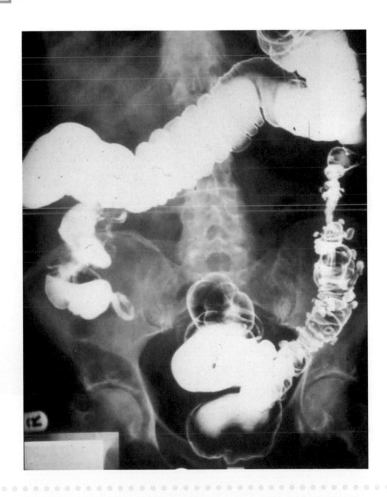

134. This elderly patient has an established history of ischaemic heart disease. She is admitted to hospital with an 8-week history of progressively worsening breathlessness. Which two of the following diagnoses would best explain the radiographic findings?

- [ ] **A** Alcoholic cardiomyopathy
- [ ] **B** Goodpasture's syndrome
- [ ] **C** Left ventricular aneurysm
- [ ] **D** Mitral valve prolapse
- [ ] **E** Restrictive cardiomyopathy
- [ ] **F** Severe aortic stenosis
- [ ] **G** Tuberculous pericarditis

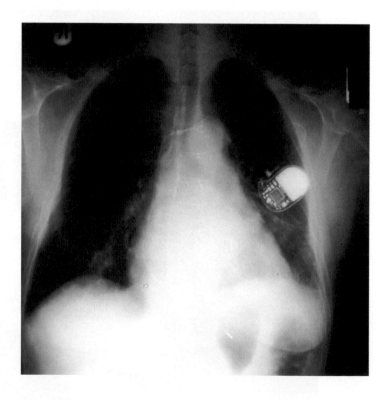

Answer on p. 180

135. This 23-year-old man is noted to have café-au-lait spots overlying his trunk and upper arms. Which one of the following complications is the patient most at risk of developing?

    A Growth hormone deficiency

    B Hyperthyroidism

    C Hypercalcaemia

    D Precocious puberty

    E Rapidly progressive renal failure

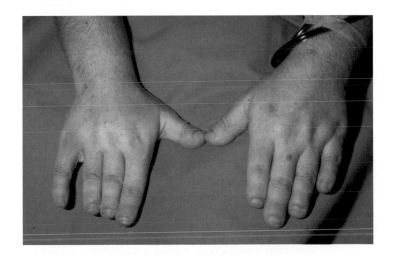

Answer on p. 180

133. **B: Chronic diverticulitis**

The appearance of multiple colonic diverticula is indicative of diverticular disease. Iron deficiency anaemia may be due to chronic blood loss from diverticular erosion into blood vessels. Other recognised complications are massive haemorrhage, localised abscess formation, chronic diverticulitis (inflammation within the diverticula), diverticular colitis (inflammation of mucosa but sparing of diverticula) and perforation, but not carcinoma. Given that diverticular disease is very common, alternative diagnoses should also be considered.

134. **A: Alcoholic cardiomyopathy, G: Tuberculous pericarditis**

Gross cardiomegaly accompanied by loss of the normal cardiac borders is highly suggestive of pericardial effusion, rather than dilated cardiomegaly or ventricular hypertrophy.

135. **B: Hyperthyroidism**

Albright's hereditary osteodystropy (AHO, McCune–Albright syndrome) describes a cluster of physical features including short stature, obesity, brachydactyly and ectopic ossifications, and endocrine disorders including precocious puberty, growth hormone excess and thyrotoxicosis. It often accompanies pseudohypoparathyroidism, with hypocalcaemia, hyperphosphataemia and high circulating parathormone concentrations (note pseudopseudohypoparathyroidism indicates AHO phenotypic features and normal end-organ responses to parathormone).

136. This 45-year-old man was diagnosed with a deep venous thrombosis of his left leg 8 years ago and an acute pulmonary thromboembolus 4 years ago, and has been taking warfarin for the past 4 years. Three weeks ago, he developed fever, cough and breathlessness on exertion, and was commenced on antibiotic therapy by his GP. Which two of the following drugs are most likely to give rise to this complication?

- ☐ **A** Amoxicillin
- ☐ **B** Ciprofloxacin
- ☐ **C** Clarithromycin
- ☐ **D** Co-amoxiclav
- ☐ **E** Flucloxacillin
- ☐ **F** Rifampicin
- ☐ **G** Trimethoprim

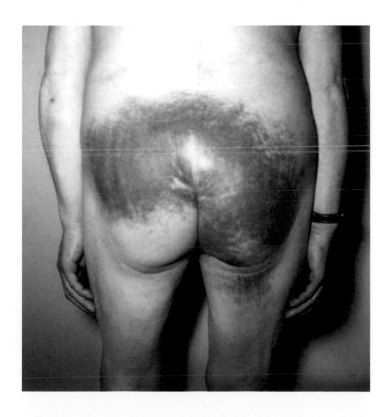

137. The following pressure traces were obtained during cardiac catheterisation studies in a 46-year-old woman. The pressure transducer is placed in the ascending aorta. What diagnosis best explains these findings?

A Aortic incompetence

B Left ventricular failure

C Mitral incompetence

D Restrictive cardiomyopathy

E Severe hypertension

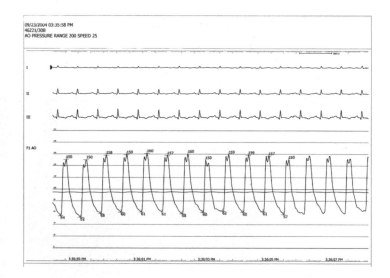

Answer on p. 184

138. A 21-year-old woman presents to the A&E department following a 999 call. She has a reduced consciousness level and smells strongly of alcohol. The ambulance crew suggest that she might have taken an overdose. Which one of the following drugs taken in overdose is likely to account for the abnormal appearance of her ECG?

- [ ] **A** Amitriptyline
- [ ] **B** Aspirin
- [ ] **C** Clozapine
- [ ] **D** Fluoxetine
- [ ] **E** Methanol

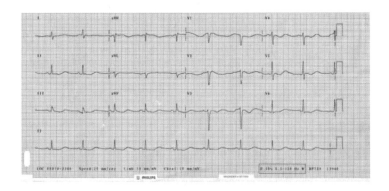

Answer on p. 184

136. B: Ciprofloxacin, C: Clarithromycin

All broad-spectrum antibiotics have the potential to enhance or reduce the absorption of warfarin to a modest degree. Ciprofloxacin, clarithromycin and erythromycin are powerful hepatic enzyme inhibitors and are most likely to significantly enhance the anticoagulant effects of warfarin. Rifampicin, a powerful enzyme inducer, might be expected to reduce the anticoagulant effect of warfarin.

137. A: Aortic incompetence

Wide pulse pressure with rapid descent of systolic pressure. A similar pattern may be seen in patients with large arterial stiffening and isolated systolic hypertension, although this would be unusual in a comparatively young patient.

138. D: Fluoxetine

Prolongation of the QT interval may be seen after overdose with selective serotonin-reuptake inhibitor (SSRI) antidepressants and antihistamines and, less commonly, after overdose with some antipsychotics, other antidepressants and other drugs, and is often a marker of increased risk of arrhythmia (including torsade de pointes).

139. This 47-year-old woman presents with an 8-day history of productive cough and mucopurulent sputum accompanied by nausea and fever symptoms. Which of the following pleural aspiration findings would be most consistent with the underlying diagnosis?

A Pleural:serum LDH ratio = 0.68

B Pleural:serum protein ratio = 0.48

C Pleural LDH 186 U/l

D Pleural protein 24 g/l

E Pleural cholesterol 3.8 mmol/l

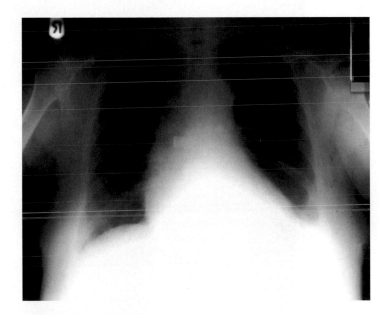

140. This 54-year-old woman is referred for investigation of progressive renal impairment. Ultrasound scan appearances of the kidneys and bladder are normal. What is the most likely underlying diagnosis?

- A Acute interstitial nephritis
- B Systemic amyloidosis
- C Systemic lupus erythematosus
- D Urate nephropathy
- E Wegener's granulomatosis

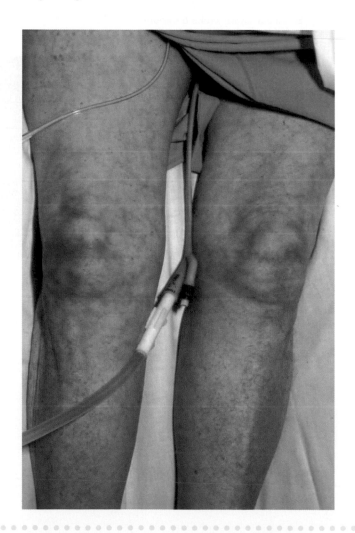

Answer on p. 188

141. This 61-year-old woman is undergoing investigation for suspected upper gastrointestinal haemorrhage. Past history includes lower limb deep vein thrombosis 9 months earlier. What diagnosis is most likely indicated by the peripheral blood film?

- **A** Chronic myeloid leukaemia
- **B** Essential thrombocythaemia
- **C** Iron deficiency anaemia
- **D** Multiple myeloma
- **E** Vitamin B$_{12}$ deficiency

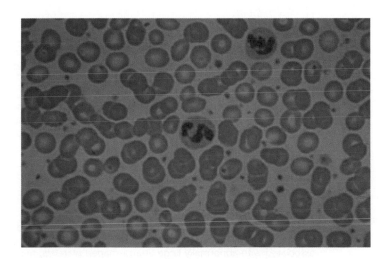

Answer on p. 188

139. **A: Pleural:serum LDH ratio = 0.68**

The history and chest radiograph are consistent with acute pneumonia and para-pneumonic effusion, which would be expected to be an exudate. Any one of Light's criteria has 98% sensitivity and 83% specificity for exudates: (i) pleural:serum protein ratio > 0.5, (ii) pleural:serum LDH ratio > 0.6, or (iii) pleural LDH > 200 U/l (two-thirds of the upper limit of normal serum values). High triglyceride and amylase concentrations suggest chylous effusion and pancreatitis-related effusion respectively.

140. **C: Systemic lupus erythematosus**

Livedo reticularis is most commonly found in young adults and is associated with bluish discoloration with a distinctive reticular pattern. It can be a benign disorder, and is also recognised as an early manifestation of systemic diseases including systemic vasculitis, rheumatoid arthritis, dermatomyositis, systemic lupus erythematosus, and cryoglobulinaemia. Sneddon's syndrome is a rare association between livedo reticularis and hypercoagulable vasculopathy.

141. **B: Essential thrombocythaemia**

Abnormally high number of platelets (that are dysfunctional), associated with abnormally large bizarre-shaped platelets, neutrophil leukocytosis and basophilia. Around 10% of cases evolve into acute leukaemia, and a further 10% of cases evolve into myelofibrosis.

142. This 58-year-old woman underwent echocardiographic investigation of intermittent dizzy spells and palpitations associated with fever symptoms and splinter haemorrhages affecting a number of nail beds. What abnormality is demonstrated by the echocardiogram (shown in M-mode view)?

A Aortic valve vegetations

B Atrial myxoma

C Mitral incompetence

D Mitral stenosis

E Ventricular aneurysm

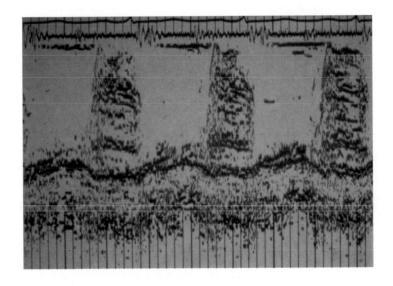

Answer on p. 192

143. This 41-year-old man is rushed to the A&E department with sudden onset of central chest pain radiating to his back. What is the most likely diagnosis?

- **A** Acute myocardial infarction
- **B** Acute pancreatitis
- **C** Acute pulmonary embolism
- **D** Oesophageal rupture
- **E** Unstable angina

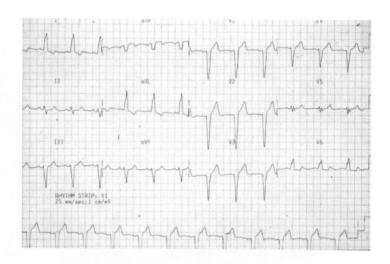

Answer on p. 192

144. A 40-year-old man with longstanding hypertension has undergone MRI scanning of the cervical and thoracic spine. He is noted to have café-au-lait spots over his limbs and trunk, and multiple soft tissue swellings over his wrists and elbows. What clinical sign would the abnormalities seen in the MRI scan be most likely to cause?

    A   Absent knee jerks

    B   Afferent papillary defect

    C   Bilateral extensor plantar responses

    D   Foot drop

    E   Tongue fasciculations

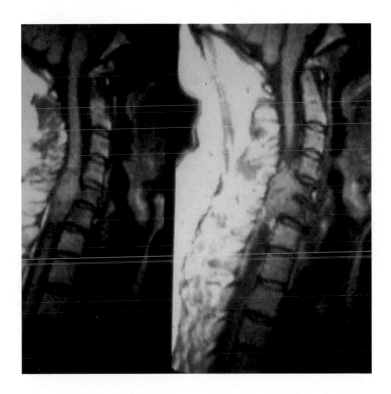

Answer on p. 192

142.   B: Atrial myxoma

Atrial myxoma is a rare condition with clinical features that may mimic infective endocarditis. There are multiple abnormal echoic signals between the mitral valve leaflets, as the tumour prolapses towards the left ventricle during diastole. AMVL = anterior mitral valve leaflet, PMVL = posterior mitral valve leaflet, 'E' (early) wave in early diastole due to passive ventricular filling, and 'a' wave in late diastole normally caused by atrial contraction.

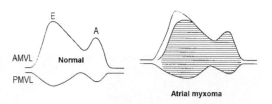

143.   A: Acute myocardial infarction

The ECG shows left bundle branch block, which can be a diagnostic feature of acute myocardial infarction. It is particularly helpful to compare with previous ECG recordings if these show previously normal conduction.

144.   C: Bilateral extensor plantar responses

This patient has neurofibromatosis, and the MRI scan demonstrates a compressive neurofibroma at the C4–C5 level, which would be expected to cause mixed upper and lower motor neurone signs in the upper limbs, and upper motor signs (increased tone, pyramidal weakness and hyperreflexia).

145. This 56-year-old patient is admitted to hospital for investigation of progressive dysphagia over the past 2 weeks. He has attended his GP 3 times in the past four months for treatment of recurrent chest infections. What abnormality does this radiological investigation most likely demonstrate?

- A Bronchiectasis
- B Cystic fibrosis
- C Mediastinal lymphadenopathy
- D Oesphago-bronchial fistula
- E Pulmonary fibrosis

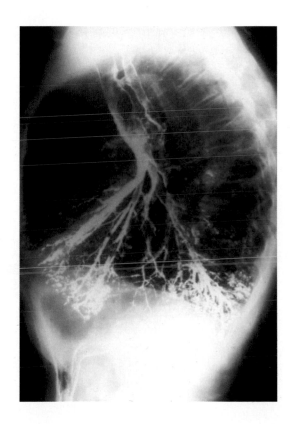

Answer on p. 196

146. This 65-year-old woman presents to hospital with sudden onset of left arm weakness and paraesthesia. Neurological examination reveals grade 4 weakness of elbow and wrist extension. Which risk factor is most likely to be responsible for her neurological symptoms?

- [ ] **A** Atrial arrhythmia
- [ ] **B** Atrial myxoma
- [ ] **C** Dilated cardiomyopathy
- [ ] **D** Hypertension
- [ ] **E** Systemic vasculitis

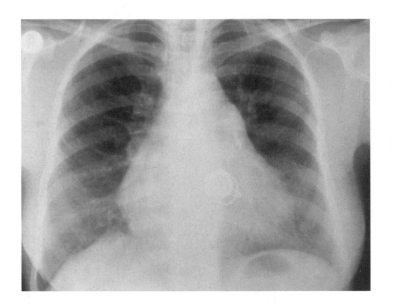

147. This 23-year-old man is referred to the general medical outpatient department for investigation of weight loss, severe sweating and fatigue. What underlying diagnosis is the most likely explanation for these abnormalities?

   A Adenocarcinoma of lung

   B HIV seroconversion illness

   C Hodgkin's lymphoma

   D Right middle lobe collapse

   E Sarcoidosis

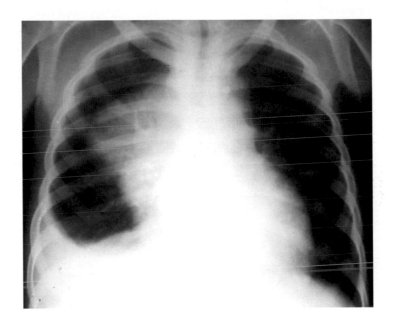

Answer on p. 196

145. **D: Oesphago-bronchial fistula**

This lateral chest radiograph with gastrograffin investigation shows obstruction to distal flow of contrast media within the proximal-to-mid oesophagus, with fistula formation and flow of contrast into the airways. This may be due to either bronchogenic or oesophageal carcinoma with local invasion.

146. **A: Atrial arrhythmia**

This patient has rheumatic valvular disease, and has previously undergone mitral valve replacement with a Starr–Edwards prosthesis. Thromboembolism is a recognised complication.

147. **C: Hodgkin's lymphoma**

Bulky enlargement of hilar lymph nodes is often a feature of underlying lymphoma. Fever, drenching night sweats and lassitude are typical 'B symptoms'.

148. This 42-year-old man is referred to the general medical outpatient department for investigation of unexplained anaemia. What is the most likely cause?

- **A** Hypothyroidism
- **B** Lead toxicity
- **C** Myelofibrosis
- **D** Sickle cell disease
- **E** Thalassaemia

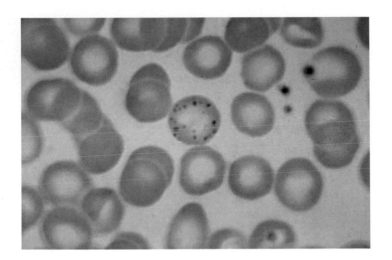

149. This patient presents with an itchy erythematous rash involving both groins. Which of the following is most likely to be an effective treatment?

- **A** Amoxicillin
- **B** Chlorpheniramine
- **C** Co-amoxiclav
- **D** Hydrocortisone
- **E** Miconazole

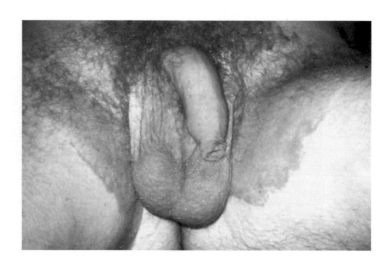

Answer on p. 200

150. This 68-year-old man is admitted to the acute medical admissions unit with palpitations and chest pain. What is the underlying cardiac rhythm?

- [ ] **A** Atrial flutter
- [ ] **B** Atrial fibrillation
- [ ] **C** Nodal tachycardia
- [ ] **D** Supraventricular tachycardia
- [ ] **E** Ventricular tachycardia

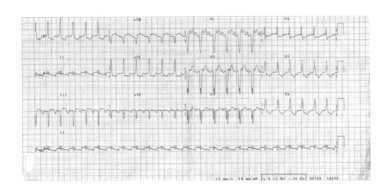

148. **B: Lead toxicity**

Basophilic stippling can be seen. Other features of chronic lead toxicity include nausea, vomiting, abdominal pain, diarrhoea or constipation, nephropathy, arthropathy ('saturnine gout'), and increased bone radio-opacification and 'lead lines' deposited in bone growth plates.

149. **E: Miconazole**

Tinea cruris is an itchy, superficial skin infection involving the groin and surrounding skin. It is caused by any one of a number of *Trichophyton* organisms, including *T. rubrum*, *T. mantagrophytes* and *T. interdigitale*.

150. **A: Atrial flutter**

Flutter activity ('F waves') are seen clearly in lead V1. Note that there is co-existent 2:1 AV nodal block and left bundle branch block, which may be caused by ischaemia due to underlying coronary artery disease and tachycardia.

INDEX

Locators refer to question numbers.

PASTEST REVISION BOOKS FOR MRCP 2

Question books

Our range of four titles for MRCP 2 provides full coverage of the MRCP 2 syllabus. Each book provides practice questions with extensive explanations to aid candidates preparing for the examination.

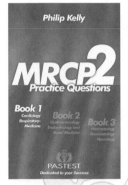

MRCP Book 1
Cardiology & Respiratory Medicine
1 904627 25 0

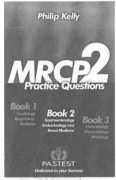

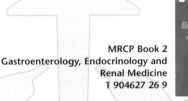

MRCP Book 2
Gastroenterology, Endocrinology and
Renal Medicine
1 904627 26 9

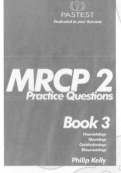

MRCP Book 3
Haematology, Rheumatology and
Neurology
1 904627 27 7

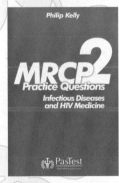

MRCP 2 Practice Questions
Infectious Diseases & HIV Medicine
1 904627 87 0

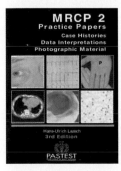

MRCP 2 Practice Papers 3rd edition
1 901198 17 0
Contains four practice papers to give candidates essential practice at questions which are similar in content and level of difficulty to the MRCP 2 examination.

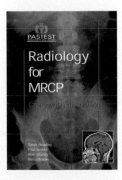

Radiology for MRCP: Cases with
discussion 2nd edition
1 901198 22 7
Contains a wide range of X-ray, MRI scans and CT scans for common cases encountered in the MRCP 2 examination.

PasTest Online Revision

Our online revision site was launched in 2004 and has been a major success with MRCP 1 and MRCS candidates. We are planning to launch MRCP 2 online revision in 2006 which will give you the opportunity for more essential practice in combination with our range of books before the examination.

Benefits of subscribing to our online revision for MRCP 2 are:

* Large data bank of questions
* Questions based on past exam themes
* Four different ways to revise: random questions, timed test, mock exam and fixed exam
* Detailed feedback on your performance compared with other users of the site
* Highly experienced doctors answering your content related queries

PasTest Online Revision is designed to suit your revision needs leading up to the exam. You can work through all the specialties within Random Questions 3–4 months prior to your exam. Once you are familiar with the entire syllabus, you can move on to the Timed Test. Here your aim should be to develop your exam strategy and techniques. You should reach this stage at least two months before the exam. Armed with your exam strategy and techniques you are ready to take Mock Exams and Fixed Exams. You should aim to be at this stage at least four weeks before your exam.

Visit www.pastestonline.co.uk to see the latest news on the launch of our online revision for MRCP 2.